T0355825

"*Ignite Your Yoga* stands as a crucial contribution to the global yoga community, offering a fresh perspective on what it means to live and embody the practice. In a world where yoga can sometimes be reduced to mere physical postures, Susanna reclaims its spiritual heritage, grounding the practice in the principles of social justice, self-awareness, and personal transformation. This book is not simply a guide or a manual—it's a call to stewardship, inviting practitioners to engage deeply with yoga's roots through sincere study, practice, and contemplation." —Kino MacGregor, author of *Accessible Ashtanga*

"*Ignite Your Yoga* is a passionate examination of the continuity of yoga from its roots to its contemporary expression. It is a skillful and rich blend of teachings that will no doubt inspire its readers to be a force for positive change on and off the mat." —Tias Little, author of *Yoga of the Subtle Body*

"A bridge between tradition and modern yoga, *Ignite Your Yoga* is a tender invitation to return to the heart of practice. With wisdom and care, Susanna Barkataki gently guides you to honor the sacred roots of this ancient practice, while empowering you to live its teachings in your modern life. Each chapter is a meditation on connection, integrity, and inclusivity, inviting you to cultivate a practice that is both deeply personal and profoundly universal. For those who seek to embody yoga's truest essence, this book will be your steady, compassionate companion on the journey." —Elena Brower, author of *Practice You*

"In *Ignite Your Yoga*, Susanna offers illumination and direction on building a yoga practice that is true and honest to yourself and to the ancient practice. She invites each reader to consider best practices and to reflect on how appropriation and misguided teachings have shaped what is known about yoga today. I am so grateful for her relentless leadership and guidance in the conversation on reclaiming yoga's roots." —Tejal Patel, Tejal Yoga

"*Ignite Your Yoga* is a heartfelt guide that seamlessly weaves tradition and modernity, inspiring a deeper commitment to yoga as a path of personal and collective transformation." —Acharya Shunya, author of *Sovereign Self*

"Susanna is the yoga leader we all need in our modern times. In *Ignite Your Yoga*, she guides us back to the beating heart of yoga, its principles, and how we can apply them to our work, leadership, home, and activism. With embodied wisdom, she shares the true diversity and beauty of what yoga can bring to our lives. This book is a must-read for those seeking to walk and share the yogic path with right-relationship, honor, and devotion to this radiant tradition." —Ann Nguyen, embodiment mentor

"This book is an invitation to step into the deeper layers of yoga, where personal growth meets collective healing. Susanna beautifully weaves together ancient wisdom and modern insight, helping you connect with yoga's true roots while making space for your own unique journey. Whether you're new to yoga or have been on the mat for years, *Ignite Your Yoga* is required reading for all who seek to show up with heart, integrity, and authenticity." —Ally Maz, author of *Girlvana*

"*Ignite Your Yoga* is an invitation to return to the sacred and the beauty that is yoga. Susanna Barkataki welcomes practitioners of all cultures and backgrounds to engage in right relationship with this practice and, ultimately, with humanity. A brilliant gift for those called to the yogic journey." —Asha Frost, author of *You Are the Medicine*

"Ignite indeed. What a gift to be reminded that we all as practitioners are responsible for caring for yoga and its future, and that our participation, whether grand or mundane, contributes to how yoga exists. Susanna expertly empowers readers around topics like reparations and cultural appropriation while providing tools for us each to live our yoga to our greatest ability." —Ava Taylor, author of *Your Yoga Business*

"This book is an act of fierce love and advocacy, and it couldn't be more urgent. Susanna is a deeply knowledgeable and inspiring guide, building on the work of generations of yoga practitioners who have used yogic philosophy to better their lives and communities. A much-needed addition to the discourse on yoga." —Charlotte Nguyen, activist, teacher, and founder of *Get Free!*

"Honoring yoga's roots, embracing the present, yoga is more than just practice—it's a deep, transformative way of living. In *Ignite Your Yoga*, Susanna Barkataki beautifully bridges ancient wisdom with the realities of today, offering a guide that is both meaningful and grounded. This book invites you to practice with deep reverence, honoring tradition while embodying integrity. It's a call to move through life with intention, creating ripples of healing and positive change, within yourself and the world around you." —Faith Hunter, author of *Spiritually Fly*

"A must-read!" —Jessamyn Stanley, author of *Every Body Yoga*

"An in depth and clear exploration of the essence of what it means to practice yoga as support for oneself while in service to others. *Ignite Your Yoga* dives into the heart of the ancient yet living tradition, carrying that joy out into the world. Uplifting and empowering." —Mary Taylor and Richard Freeman, authors of *Feeling Happy*

"Susanna brings the deep roots, key principles, and ethics of yoga to 'the West' in an accessible, digestible format that is both actionable and immediately impactful. This book is a gift for all who are ready to learn from an authentic source how yoga can not only improve your daily life but also deepen your life purpose and contribute to collective healing. Everyone who cares about personal and collective well-being and peace should read this book." —Emily Anne Brant, Indigenous Wisdom Keeper

"I'm so happy Susanna Barkataki has written this book for the world! Her vision, emphasizing the impact of yoga on our lives and mental health, is so timely. Even better, she dares to be authentic about the tradition and practice of yoga. The teachings she's kind enough to broach allow every single one of us to learn *at least* one new thing about ourselves through the power of yoga." —Mychal Threets, Mychal the Librarian

"*Ignite Your Yoga* serves as a guide for these times. Susanna provides us with practices that can help spiritually root us and guide us back to each other, our bodies, and restoring harmony and balance. And she does all this while honoring the lineage of yoga and without spiritually bypassing the oppressive systems we live in. In essence, she gifts us a guide for embodying true spirituality to hold us as we navigate this current paradigm and birth the new one." —Dr. Rocio Rosales Meza, Seer and Medicine Woman

"A must-read book for yogis who are looking to deepen and embody their practice with appreciation, not appropriation. An important book for these times, I can't recommend it enough." —Rebecca Campbell, author of *Your Soul Had a Dream, Your Life Is It*

"*Ignite Your Yoga* should be in every modern Western yoga practitioner's hands; indeed, it's one I wish I had when I was starting my own practice. Barkataki's voice is gentle and compassionate, even as it gives us the critical challenge of taking our yoga practice beyond mere fitness and self-help, and returning it to its rightful roots: tradition, ethics, and a unified self-world sense. I am confident that this book will not only 'ignite' more powerful yoga practices but also more peace, kindness, and collective action across the world." —Simone Seol, founder of HOME

IGNITE YOUR YOGA

HOW TO LIVE, PRACTICE, AND TEACH AS AN AUTHENTIC YOGA STEWARD

SUSANNA BARKATAKI

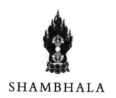

SHAMBHALA

Shambhala Publications, Inc.
2129 13th Street
Boulder, Colorado 80302
www.shambhala.com

© 2025 by Susanna Barkataki

Cover art: vika_k/Adobe Stock
Cover design: Daniel Urban-Brown
Interior design: Gopa & Ted2, Inc

All rights reserved. No part of this book may be reproduced in any form or by any means, electronic or mechanical, including photocopying, recording, or by any information storage and retrieval system, without permission in writing from the publisher.

9 8 7 6 5 4 3 2 1

First Edition
Printed in the United States of America

Shambhala Publications makes every effort to print on acid-free, recycled paper. Shambhala Publications is distributed worldwide by Penguin Random House, Inc., and its subsidiaries.

Library of Congress Cataloging-in-Publication Data
Names: Barkataki, Susanna, author.
Title: Ignite your yoga: how to live, practice, and teach as an authentic yoga steward / Susanna Barkataki.
Description: First edition. | Boulder, Colorado: Shambhala Publications, Inc., [2025] | Includes bibliographical references. |
Identifiers: LCCN 2024030690 | ISBN 9781611809947 (trade paperback; acid-free paper)
Subjects: LCSH: Yoga.
Classification: LCC B132.Y6 B343 2025 | DDC 204/.36–dc23/eng/20240813
LC record available at https://lccn.loc.gov/2024030690

Contents

Beginning Invocation

ॐ सह नाववतु ।
सह नौ भुनक्तु ।
सह वीर्यं करवावहै ।
तेजस्वि नावधीतमस्तु मा विद्विषावहै ।
ॐ शान्तिः शान्तिः शान्तिः ॥

OM SAHANA VAVATU

SAHANAU BHUNAKTU

SAHAVIRYAM KARAVAVAHAI

TEJASVINA VADHITA MASTU MA VIDVISHAVAHAI

OM SHANTI SHANTI SHANTIHI

May we both be nourished.
May we both be protected.
May we work together with great energy.
May our studies be enlightening.
May there be no enmity between us.

Peace in body, mind, and spirit. Peace in all three realms.

From *Krishna Yajurveda Taittiriya Upanishad*;[1] this chant is often shared at the start of a school class or at the beginning of a yoga practice to send nourishing energy for learning together on this spiritual journey with yoga.

Acknowledgments

I WANT TO BEGIN with a deep bow to honor the land and the roots of the sacred tradition of yoga and all the yogis from India—from Shiva to Patanjali—who have practiced and taught so that we can benefit today. I honor and thank every single teacher and student who has brought me here.

I wouldn't be who I am today without the wisdom and work of so many who came before me.

FAMILY AND PERSONAL SUPPORT

Thank you to my parents, Shan and Cathy Barkataki, for everything. Your support of this path is immeasurable. Huge gratitude to Shan for sharing traditions and to Cathy, for reading, re-reading, and editing this manuscript. You are both amazing, and I'm so grateful to be your daughter.

Thank you to my loves Eran and Kailash James. Eran, your unwavering support, love, and patience have been my rock throughout this journey. Your belief in me has given me strength during the toughest times. Kailash, your joy and curiosity inspire me daily and remind me of the importance of pursuing one's passions with an open heart.

Special thanks to my family and friends, whose joy, emotional support, and understanding were crucial in helping me navigate the challenges of this project. Your patience and encouragement kept me inspired. I can't name all of you, but you know who you are!

Thank you to all the incredible yoga lovers, practitioners, teachers, and creators at Yoke Yoga who guided this book. What a joy to explore the heart of yoga in bite-size, social, free, and fun ways that are also so diverse and accessible. You might come for the flexibility, but you stayed for the spiritual journey. And that means everything.

Huge bows of gratitude to all of the students in Embody Yoga's Roots Yoga Teacher Training 200 and 300 Hour as well as Yoga Class Curator, Teach Yoga to Millions, and Embrace Yoga's Roots Courses. We create the most amazing lifelong learning communities! Your questions and insights always keep me on my toes and connected to my heart.

I bow to you, dear reader.

PROFESSIONAL SUPPORT

Linda Sparrowe, your guidance from conception to development aided the writing of this book. Our times together were more than writing and became a part of life with your unwavering guidance, insightful feedback, and continuous encouragement throughout the research process. Your expertise and dedication were instrumental in shaping this project.

Thanks too to: Beth Frankl, for inviting me into the Shambhala family and believing in this vision; incredible editors Breanna Locke and Emily Wichland; and the whole publishing team at Shambhala.

And also to Tiwanna Shipp, Linda Lopes, Trish Hosein, Juliana Mirielles, Sunaina Rangnekar, and M Camelia for making the magic at Ignite and Yoke Yoga.

TEACHERS AND INFLUENCES

My first teachers: my parents and family in Assam and Bengal, particularly Prasanta Barkataki, Cathy Barkataki, and Maya Bhaumik, who taught me the essence of everything I've learned and showed me that our traditions are not separate from our lives. Shankarji in the Shankaracharya tradition, Kabirji, Dr. Vandana Shiva, Satish Kumar, H. H. the Dalai Lama, A. T. Ariyaratne, Thich Nhat Hanh,

Eisha Mason, Dr. Rev Lawson, Michele Benzamin-Miki, and many others.

I'm deeply grateful to study and practice yoga and Ayurveda in the tradition of engaged Hatha Yoga in the Shankaracharya tradition.

Honoring the Land and Elements

I bow to the earth and elements that make up all life: the stars, sky, sun, moon, and all the elements—earth, water, fire, air, and space.

I am so grateful for my teachers and all the early practitioners of the yogic path of liberation; you shine like a path of stars lighting up the sky of liberation.

May the fruits of this practice benefit all beings.

A deep bow to you. OM SHANTI SHANTI SHANTI.

Introduction

I **BELIEVE IN YOGA** like I believe in the power of love. It is my path, my practice, and my dharma. I was born into the yoga tradition, and I made a conscious choice to pursue it deeply. I feel its presence within my heart and soul. I know from the letters I receive, the conversations I've had, and the trainings I lead that many of you feel the same way and are curious about the many ways to embody yoga in your life. I feel this. I really do. So, I wrote *Ignite Your Yoga* to explore yoga as a spiritual practice; to investigate the many ways each of us can say *yes* to this ancient tradition as a vehicle for personal, social, and collective liberation. I often think of yoga as *practical*, in-the-world spirituality that provides the tools we need to engage with ourselves, each other, and the planet with clarity, confidence, and compassion. Because of that, it has the power to create complete and total transformation.

If you've been practicing for any length of time, you may already know that the word *yoga* means "union"—union with self and with others. It is a union that embraces paradox. This isn't a union that erases differences but celebrates and honors them. It's that sense of union that can be born even out of separation. An awareness of connection with your body, breath, mind, and heart that invites you to explore your deepest self, an inner knowing, and maybe even hear a whisper of meaning and purpose. In saying yes to this exploration, you are also choosing to turn toward the heart of yoga.

Yoga also means union with others, offering a deep sense of kinship that allows you to listen to someone's heart and see them in their fullest potential—and to receive the gift of being fully seen and held yourself.

Yoga is union with community, or sangha—your chosen spiritual family in which you join with a group of people united by common values, causes, hobbies, passions, or circumstances where shared humanity and mutual understanding can emerge.

Yoga is union that creates liberation for all, reminding you that though we show up in an infinite array of experiences, there is no separation between you and other beings. No one can be free until all beings are free.

Yoga is about not just union or oneness but also understanding and embodying our unique experience so fully that we are completely whole within ourselves. There are many paths to a deeper understanding of yoga. Wherever you are on your path, from beginner to very experienced, you can read this book and let it and yoga change you. We are always students on this path. The more you practice, the deeper you go. The deeper you commit, the more you are changed.

Every time I open a yoga text, talk with colleagues, or visit my extended family in India and spend time with my teachers there, I'm reminded that our understanding of "yoga as truth and union" is often quite different from in the West. In India, and for some of us in the diaspora, yoga is what connects us to all of life. It's something that is woven into the very fabric of our being, and there are myriad ways to practice it. It is the way we come together with our families, friends, and communities; the way we serve others. There's a context of spiritual consciousness and collective care, though historically and currently people have always practiced in different ways.

In the West we sometimes miss this context. As someone born at the intersection of both worlds—with an Indian father and British mother—the contrast between cultures has been evident my whole life. I made the commitment to dive deeper into my Indian heritage through study and practice. Much of my work is both a personal and a social attempt at unity—creating a bridge between worlds.

Often, as it is practiced in the West, yoga is what allows us to connect to ourselves, to get *away from* life, from the very real, impactful, and often deeply uncomfortable issues going on "out there." It's something we can do to forget about our troubles for a while. Something we can do to strengthen our bodies and calm our nervous systems. By the time we conclude our practice session, we feel a little better about ourselves. That's not to say that the connection we feel to our bodies and hearts is not a true yogic connection. It absolutely is. It's just that when yoga happens on our mats behind closed doors, it may paradoxically serve to create more separation than connection. How? By prioritizing self-care over collective care, those who can afford to take classes over those who cannot, the desire to look and feel better over the desire to be and do better. It sometimes becomes a means of praying away problems, sending love and light out into a world that needs engagement, without actually having to *engage* ourselves. As a result, hundreds of thousands of practitioners know plenty about the third limb of yoga—maybe even the fourth— but next to nothing about how yoga prepares us all for a life of compassionate service.

In spite of all this, I'm hopeful. Why? Because with yoga it is not a forced choice. We can care for ourselves while caring for the world, and both are enhanced by doing the other. I've already begun to notice a change. Rather than avoiding *dukkha*—the immense suffering in the world—more yoga practitioners are asking how they can utilize their practice to address their own and others' suffering and create liberation. Many are becoming more aware of this expanded way of living yoga. Conversations are happening in studios and online, before class and after hours, as teachers and students begin to grapple with how to expand their knowledge in order to bring the true wisdom of yoga into their lives and the lives of others. The success of my first book, *Embrace Yoga's Roots: Courageous Ways to Deepen Your Yoga Practice*, is a testament to the importance of these discussions and has guided and encouraged many of them. Students are reading more and insisting that their studios—and their teacher-training programs—bring cultural representation and decolonize their bookshelves and reading lists. We see yoga teachers unionizing and yoga centers prioritizing wisdom, action, reflection, and social change. Things are happening!

It does my heart good to see so many leaning into the heart of yoga, working to make yoga more accessible and integrated. Teachers with diverse experiences, abilities, body types, colors, and cultures are showing up on the covers of magazines and, more importantly, in classrooms, practice spaces, and communities all over. Practitioners are learning that they don't have to be able to touch their toes or wear fancy yoga clothes to have a full, well-rounded practice. Teacher-training programs are inviting more of us in as guest presenters to provide a deeper historical, cultural, and spiritual context. Teachers and practitioners are experiencing yoga in and beyond asana and exploring the fullness of all that yoga has to offer.

However, a full, expansive yoga practice is still greatly misunderstood in the West. If we intend to connect yoga to its true essence and practice in ways relevant to relieving our own suffering and the suffering of others, we've got more work to do. We must learn to apply it to our lives moment to moment. It's no longer a question of why; it's a question of how. How do we move from centering the individual, which fosters separation and inequity, to honoring the collective, which encourages interconnectedness and compassionate action? How can we see that our obsession with our own physical health and well-being comes at the expense of the health and well-being of others?

I believe the answer lies first and foremost in understanding that yoga is not something we *do* but rather something we *are*. Yoga is at its core a spiritual practice; it reminds us that our liberation and joy are inextricably linked to the liberation and joy of all beings. When we embrace the fullness of yoga, we become yoga stewards— yoga teachers and students who live our lives from the yogic lens of union and interconnection. To be a yoga steward means that we consciously choose to preserve the teachings of yoga in everything we do.

Of course, that can't happen unless we know *what* we're preserving and *how* to preserve it—and equally important, what we need to leave behind. That's why I wrote this book. Yoga is a *living* tradition, one that evolves to meet the culture and context it finds itself in. Many aspects of yoga have stood the test of time for thousands of years; practices that support individual and collective liberation, that bring ease and clarity to the body and mind; practices that help us live our lives in integrity, unity, and love. This is the yoga we're talking about.

There are also aspects of the tradition that are patriarchal, normative, caste oppressive, misogynistic, and that otherwise condone harmful ideas and acts of oppression—ideas and practices that reflect more on the customs, norms, and behaviors of a particular time and place than on yoga itself. It is up to us as yoga stewards to recognize and acknowledge what continues to oppress and create harm, and actively work to dismantle that—first within ourselves and then in our relationships, communities, and beyond. Only then can we return to the heart of the practice, the true essence of yoga, so that it can take its rightful place in the collective wellness arena and bring us the peace, healing, and transcendence that a full yoga experience offers.

How to Use This Book

Ignite Your Yoga is a guidebook for your authentic spiritual journey. In it you'll find suggestions on how to live yogic values in your personal life and how to assume a leadership role on the mat, in your relationships, and in your work in the world. You'll get practical tools for spiritual connection, which can help you walk the path of a yoga steward and move into true leadership in ways that honor and support the teachings of this ancient practice. If you would like a complimentary guided version of some of the practices and meditations in this book, download it at IgniteYourYoga.com.

Within the pages of this book—and through the work I do—I invite all of us to commit to yoga as a spiritual practice, a personal sadhana, and to experience it as a system of personal, collective, and social transformation. I want teachers to learn how to offer up the tradition itself as a means of addressing the sadness, fear, and separation within the individual, as well as a means of creating a more unified and equitable world. We can only do this if those of us who have benefited from this practice commit wholeheartedly to preserving the tradition by how we practice it, live it, and take it out into the world.

I invite you to read the chapters in *Ignite Your Yoga* sequentially the first time through. We often say yoga is not yoga until it's personal. And I believe that. No one can know yoga without first experiencing it in their body, mind, and heart. So that's where the book begins—as an invitation to preserve the teachings through your personal practice.

I also believe that yoga is not yoga until we give it away. You may reap the benefits of yoga as spiritual practice and yet you don't own them. You get to share them with others—those you love, those you struggle with, even those you'd rather avoid altogether. How do you do that? By embodying yoga in all that you are and all that you do. In part 1, I lay a foundation and ground for our practice. In part 2, we bring yoga into our lives as I share many more personal stories, helpful teachings, tools, and practices that can help you preserve the teachings through how you show up in relationships, show up in service, and create positive change in the world—as an agent of spiritual possibility.

Part 1: Centering the Tradition

It's important to know what we are and are not preserving before we commit to the spiritual path of a yoga steward. So, this first section focuses on the *essence* of yoga as outlined by the sage Patanjali in the Yoga Sutras. We take time to define the eight limbs—including the *yamas* and *niyamas* (how we care for others and for ourselves)—in ways that may feel familiar to you as well as in ways that may surprise you. This sets the stage for the rest of the book as we look at yoga through the lens of personal practice, relationships, compassionate service, and social change.

Part 2: Heeding the Sadhaka's Call

A *sadhaka* is one devoted to yoga as spiritual practice; one whose everyday life is infused with and informed by yoga's deeper teachings. This section explores what that means and invites you to listen to the call to yoga and commit to it fully—within yourself, in your personal relationships, and in your work in the world. I'll admit making such a commitment is not always easy—especially when life feels full of obligations. So, to guide you in such an inquiry, I've offered eight steps along the path of a sadhaka or yoga steward that have helped me in my practice. These steps come from foundational texts such as the *Hatha Yoga Pradipika*, though I've brought them into our modern world so they apply to our lives. They are not prescriptive. They are descriptive of skills, tools, and ways of being we can develop as we explore our yoga practice. Like any spiritual path, of course, this one is not linear; it's more like a spiral, perhaps even a labyrinth—something you can return to at different times and at various stages in your life and practice.

It's not enough, of course, to heed the call within the confines of your mat or cushion. Because this is what I know to be true: *you can't live what you don't practice*, and *you can't offer others what you don't live.* So, embedded in each step are ways to move the dial from how to *embody* the tradition to how to *live* it daily; to take what you've learned on your mat and move it into your relationships—with your partner, parents, children, work colleagues, or communities.

The problems of our time cannot be solved with logic alone. We need heartfelt solutions for an interwoven humanity, ways of thinking about and solving problems that don't just keep our interconnectedness in mind but truly embody it. As sadhakas on the path, we are agents of spiritual possibility—people actively working to disrupt cynicism, apathy, and inaction. I unpack what that means and how to choose service that aligns with your dharma, the deeper meaning of your life and your sacred purpose in the world.

As we move into conscious leadership, we do it with purpose, step by step, making incremental changes. Whether we are tackling huge issues or taking small steps, when we make changes in our personal practice and in how we live it, those changes have an effect in making the world a better place. And we look at the question: How can we preserve the essence of yoga, serve in a yogic way, and at the same time disrupt and dismantle the harm done historically and currently while creating change we truly believe in?

Throughout the book you'll hear from some incredible yoga sadhakas who inspire me with all the ways they are practicing, living, and leading with yoga. Keep an eye out for those "Sadhakas Speak" moments to pause, breathe, and take in the wisdom from the many yogic lineage keepers. The very last "Sadhakas Speak" might just be a surprise!

I wrote this book for those who are ready to cast aside the watered-down versions of yoga and connect to the depth of what this ancient practice has to offer. I wrote this book for anyone who has ever stepped on a mat; anyone who is teaching yoga, starting a yoga clothing brand, running a studio, or seeking to share yoga with their classrooms or their children; anyone who longs to become intimately connected to the roots of yoga, to feel the heart and soul of yoga—and then take it out into the world for the benefit of all beings.

Part One
Centering the Tradition

The foreigners have stolen all the skills and knowledge and treasures of Mother India, either right in front of us or in a hidden way. They pretend that they have discovered all this by themselves, bundle it together, and then bring it back here as though doing us a favour and in exchange take all the money and things we have saved up for our family's welfare. After some time passes, they will try and do the same thing with yogavidya.

KRISHNAMACHARYA

Yoga Stewardship

IN THE HEART OF a city, where whispers of wisdom float on chants through the busy streets, there was a revered sannyasi known to be a guardian of the sacred teachings. He taught anyone—be they Muslim, traveler, Dalit, young, or old. He stewarded and shared yogic wisdom with all who were open to learning. This yogi's name was Shankar, after his beloved lineage teacher Sri Adi Shankara-charya, and he had just emerged from a decade of solitary retreat. He embodied the essence of yoga stewardship, a commitment to nurturing and sharing the spiritual, ethical, and practical aspects of yoga with integrity and love. "In the act of living yoga, we stew-ard it. We illuminate the path for others, just as the stars light the night sky," he would often say in encouragement. He implored us to practice, live, and steward yoga within our own communities. I saw how his life was a testament to the power of serving as a bridge between the ancient wisdom of yoga and modern seekers like me, guiding us through the practices of asana, meditation, and selfless service. He taught that true yoga stewardship means not just prac-ticing on the mat but living yoga in every moment, every breath, and every interaction. By doing so, we become beacons of light and love, inspiring others to embark on their own journey of discovery and transformation. We called him Shankarji as a sign of respect. His mission reminds us that in the heart of yoga stewardship lies the call to nurture our connection to the self, others, and the world around us, embodying the profound unity that yoga teaches.

Yoga deepens within us when we commit to it as our sadhana, or spiritual practice. Yoga comes alive when we become a vessel for the expression of unity and agree to nurture its gifts and share them with the utmost respect; when we begin to understand that through yoga we can awaken to our true nature; that it can inform and enrich our sense of self and our place in the world.

You don't have to have a weekly schedule of *vinyasa* flow classes to commit to yoga stewardship, although you might. You don't have to call yourself a yoga teacher, although that's possible too. Being a yoga steward means that you are steeped in the practice and that you share it naturally—and in an accessible way—through the qualities you embody. You preserve the tradition in the way you live it because you know that yoga has the power to change minds and hearts—and transform lives. So, you may be stewarding yoga through your work as an accountant, teacher, bus driver, parent, or engineer at NASA working to launch rockets into space. Remember, yoga isn't something you do, it's something you are. The focus is less on *what* you do than on *how* you do it. You show up in all areas of your life *in a yogic way*.

Yoga stewardship asks that you put this ancient practice into its proper cultural and historical context—from its roots to modern day. That means you stay open to inquiring about and learning yoga history. But it doesn't mean that you view it through rose-colored glasses. Stewardship requires that you uncover, acknowledge, and then work to repair the harm yoga has caused throughout the millennia—and continues to do today. And, at the same time, that you bring forth practices that center individual and collective liberation and that come from a place of love.

How Can Yoga Stewardship Address Cultural Appropriation?

Let's address cultural appropriation as this might be a topic on your mind and heart as it is for so many seeking to embrace the heart of what yoga offers us. Deciding what to honor within the yoga tradition and what to leave behind or work to dismantle can be tricky for sure. Is it even possible to honor and appreciate certain teachings and aspects of a tradition and not others—without participating in cultural appropriation? I believe it is. But before diving into how to do that, I'd like to first get clear on the difference between appropriation and appreciation.

Cultural Appropriation

Cultural appropriation happens when a dominant group adopts, benefits from, shares, and even exploits the customs, practices, ideas, social and spiritual knowledge of another, often subordinate group of people—without considering the source, origins, or people of that culture. When that happens, it exacerbates and highlights systemic, often global, inequities. It can often cause irreparable harm across social institutions and political, economic, social, spiritual, and cultural worlds.

Cultural appropriation always involves two criteria: power inequity and harm. Inequity of power is always structural, such as with colonization, where one group holds power over another. The harm can be personal, interpersonal, systemic, cultural, political, or spiritual. We see examples of cultural appropriation all the time in Western yoga circles. Studio owners, yoga teachers, and even students don't always realize they've done anything wrong. They might think they're being innovative, adding a little bit of "unique" or "Eastern" flair to their style. They may even think they've included a design element that *honors* the tradition when they're actually doing the opposite. For example, when I see an OM symbol, a sign of unity and spiritual transcendence, painted on a yoga studio floor where it will be stepped on, or hanging upside down and crooked on a wall, I feel it in my gut. The disrespect cuts like a knife. It's like my whole culture and experience is being trivialized at best, or even erased. And saying "But I didn't mean to hurt anyone" doesn't eliminate or soften the impact of the harm they've caused. This harm happens within a context of continual exploitation of one group by another. To truly practice yoga requires us to be conscious and intentional about our actions, truthfully acknowledging the impact of those actions on others and working to repair the damage.

I think it's important to pause for a moment and recognize that cultural appropriation is not confined to modern-day yoga practitioners—although it is certainly a problem in the West. We often talk about Western appropriation of yoga, but cultural appropriation is more complex than that and began far earlier. Yoga has long been co-opted and adulterated for purposes of domination by those in power in South Asia. A prime example is the Brahminical patriarchy's appropriation of the earth-based yoga traditions, which were for and from the people. It is important to distinguish Brahminical patriarchy from *Brahmanism*, an ancient religious tradition that was the precursor to Hinduism. Brahmanism is rooted in the Vedic texts and emphasizes the worship of Brahman, the ultimate reality or universal spirit in Hindu philosophy. It can also refer to the broad cultural religious and philosophical practices tied to the Vedic system beyond the caste system. However, a small and increasingly powerful subsection of society codified power and control over these practices under the name of Brahminical patriarchy. For centuries this appropriation, along with protest and dissension, actions and policies, separated and punished those who were not part of the normative elite. Such appropriation continues unabated today. Caste apartheid leveled against Dalit people—in India and in the West—is a particularly violent and heinous example of appropriation by Brahminical patriarchal social structures that has long resulted in oppression and genocide. In her groundbreaking book *The Trauma of Caste: A Dalit Feminist Meditation on Survivorship, Healing, and Abolition*, the transmedia artist, futurist, and Dalit activist Thenmozhi Soundararajan explains,

> People in the West need to know that most of the spiritual, intellectual, and cultural products of South Asia are tainted by Brahmanism. What may have offered you liberation and healing also causes caste-oppressed people to suffer. You don't have to give up those practices or con-

cepts, but the call is to be intentional and acknowledge the caste harm.[1]

I asked Soundararajan to speak more about her work to a group of us in an online workshop. What was eye-opening to many was how the Brahminical patriarchy appropriated the yogic tradition as its own, including its spiritual texts and language—and interpreted it to solidify its power. It forbade Dalit people, known in Brahmanism as the "untouchable" caste, to speak, read, or even hear Sanskrit, which was the language in which the laws of their fate are written. Dalits were not even allowed to have any relationship with a higher being because they were "considered spiritually defiling before God," Thenmozhi explained. It can be challenging to witness how yoga has been used out of alignment with its own principles to exclude and oppress. As we reclaim the roots of yoga, it is part of honoring the original inclusive, earth-based practices like Bhramanism and other pre-Vedic yoga practices. We can think critically about the root values we want to bring forward, such as those of liberation, truth, and non-harm.

There are many parallels between appropriation of yoga in India and the appropriation of yoga in the West. Both are examples of how cultural appropriation by a dominant culture can harm those they oppress. We see this far too often in studios throughout the West that center and elevate a normative dominant culture experience at the expense of Black, Brown, South Asian, and Indigenous populations; LGBTQ+ folks; and people with disabilities, to name a few. As yoga stewards, we are obligated—indeed, it is part of our dharmic commitment—to work toward calling out and abolishing such systems of oppression and becoming stewards of inclusion and healing. We will talk more about what it means in practical terms in part 2.

From Guilt to Cultural Care and Connection

::

It's common when learning about cultural appropriation to feel frustrated, grieving, or guilty about our thoughts, words, and actions. The awareness of harm can give rise to a sense that we've done something wrong or that wrongs have been done. That's not a bad thing if it helps us realize where and how we or others may have erred and where and how we can make changes. However, it is not helpful—or pleasant—to stay stuck in guilt and remorse. It is so important to move through the guilt and grief to creativity and care! How can we do this? Acknowledge the guilt, anger, or grief. Acknowledge the harm. And recognize that by doing so, you show your care and that you are willing to grow and make changes. And then . . . make those changes! Celebrate yourself along the way.

Cultural appreciation and connection are a beautiful process.

Cultural Appreciation and Connection

Whereas appropriation is choosing aspects of another culture that will justify our own behaviors—and often solidify our power over others—cultural appreciation is the desire to connect with cultures different from our own from the *inside out*. It respects the codes, mores, values, and practices of the culture. It often happens when we value, enjoy, and uplift the culture of origin. Cultural appreciation involves two criteria that are the exact opposite of what creates appropriation. When we appreciate, we seek to restore the balance of power. Instead of harm, we seek to practice non-harm and care:

- **Power balancing.** We can practice cultural appreciation when we look at the imbalance of power and address it.

When we share social location or use our privilege or advantage to uplift or support an under-resourced person or group of people, we are balancing power. For example, when caste-privileged folks work toward caste abolition, or when white Western folks uplift Desis and other South Asians in yoga spaces by sharing their books, workshops, and pointing to their cultural knowledge. Working with power in this way is part of working with *Shakti* (life force/power) in yoga. Practicing to own, honor, and equalize power is part of the tools that a full, expansive yoga practice cultivates.

- **Non-harm (ahimsa).** Practicing cultural appreciation rather than appropriation begins by embodying the yogic principle of ahimsa (non-harm). Ahimsa is when we actively work to reduce or mitigate harm. It is the consideration, care, and respect we give when we commit to learning about and uplifting the source culture and those who often don't receive support. This can include financial, social, political, emotional, and cultural care and support. For example, if a caste-privileged South Asian is teaching yoga, an act of ahimsa might mean they share a caste nondiscrimination statement at the beginning of each class and perhaps donate a percentage of the profits they make to folks and organizations working for caste equity and abolition. Similarly, a yoga studio or yoga teacher-training program run by white folks could include books by South Asian authors as required reading; bring in South Asian guest teachers; and work to cite sources and learn cultural elements to care for the practice.

So, the question remains: Is it possible to preserve some but not all of the ancient teachings without committing cultural appropriation? I believe it is. In fact, I believe we as yoga stewards have an opportunity to learn and pass along the sacred wisdom of yoga, which has worked for thousands of years to reduce suffering and increase peace—and to abolish the harmful practices that have caused pain and separation. To do that, we must carefully consider the aspects of yoga we want to foster and nurture, and which aspects we don't. We can be mindful of leaving aside patriarchy and oppression while we bring in care for cultural issues, inclusion, and diversity.

Many different lineages, styles, schools, and traditions—ancient and contemporary—offer their own version of the yogic path toward liberation. As far back as 2500 B.C.E., exploration of the divine, spirit, and deep inquiry into the self was appreciated, understood, and supported. We know this because during this time, despite the advancements in comfort and lifestyle, many folks left a newly developing civilization in the Indus Valley to seek a deeper, truer kind of peace and inner satisfaction. These sannyasins (renunciates) formed a kind of forest monastic culture of various and diverse practices intent on figuring out how to relieve suffering and find fulfillment and joy. They were in relationship with the villages and cities around them and were often taken care of and fed by local villagers. These early seekers of truth found a system—a set of processes and practices—that led them into union with themselves, their true nature, the natural world, and divine consciousness. They called this system "yoga."

The alternative to cultural appropriation is often creativity. Creativity allows us to tune in to the world around us, our own historical roots, our relationships, the earth, the land, and all people. From this place of connection we are much more often going to heal rather than harm. There has never been just one way to practice yoga. There have always been many ways, not unlike there are today. Today we may argue over classical practices or more contemporary applications, such as how to be trauma informed. Debate is not new for yoga. Throughout its thousands-year-long history, lively debates ensued among what we might call practitioner-scholars as well as whole schools and lineages discussing the foundational tenets they believed would lead to liberation. There are those who believe and teach that personal liberation comes through complete detachment from the senses and the world; and those who believe and practice yoga in connection with others to find liberation. Each path respects one another, though their approaches to liberation differ. This is still true today. We even see some of these differences in how the limbs of yoga are articulated. There were six limbs of yoga named at first, and then eight pieces of the yoga pie that led to well-being. The two pieces that were added later were the yamas and niyamas—the ethical and personal codes of yoga, clearly so needed in ancient and modern times. The broad and far-reaching multiplicity of yoga practices historically gives us a comprehensive framework to bring into our present day.

What's next is for us to fold these pieces into our lives. There are many ways into a deeper understanding of yoga. Ancient texts such as the Yoga Sutras of Patanjali, the Bhagavad Gita, the Upanishads, and the *Hatha Yoga Pradipika*, when used properly, can be indispensable guides that can help us get to know ourselves, honor our relationships, and care for and serve others. Although there are many more classical texts and paths we could focus on, for our purposes here, it's important to emphasize yoga practices that make ethical considerations practical and possible in our modern world. When my teacher Shankarji guided me to share yogic ethics in the West, he told me to "take these practices and bring them where they are needed most. The West *needs* yogic ethics." I've focused on Raja Yoga, as laid out in the Yoga Sutras of Patanjali,[2] specifically the eight limbs of yoga that move us toward personal and collective liberation and transformation. The first four limbs—the yamas, niyamas, asana, and pranayama—are more external practices, and we should do them simultaneously (chapters 2, 3, 4 and 5). The last three—dharana, dhyana, and samadhi—are the internal practices, and we should do them sequentially (chapters 7, 8, and 9). *Pratyahara*, the fifth limb, is the bridge between the external and internal practices (chapter 6). Every limb is grounded in love and non-harming (ahimsa), in truth and justice (*satya*), and in our connection to the divine essence (*ishvara pranidhana*). Anything not grounded in love and non-harm, truth and justice, is an imposter that might lead us away from the heart of our yoga practice.

SADHAKAS SPEAK: SUNAINA RANGNEKAR

::

My sadhana feels like letting go of perfection and looks like allowing my feelings to show. Crying to make room. Doing my makeup to my favorite tunes. Alignment of the breath to my body—anything that creates more flow. My sadhana is a group mantra with my community and focused tantra with my partner(s). It's being gentle with myself when I miss a day. It's dream journaling when I first awake and watching the seeds of my life grow into buds, then grow into flowers—all of which I planted with devotion to Narayana. It's the act of picking those flowers, arranging them on my altar as offerings to my (tr)ancestors. It's releasing the outcome. It's noticing the cycles of the seasons and adjusting my sleep, food, and rituals to match. It's speaking my affirmations out loud to myself each day, feeling the vibration of those words resonate through my body. My sadhana is speaking Tamil as often as possible, especially to my Patti. In autonomy, my sadhana is my daily lived experience. It is the embodiment of all parts of my unconscious and conscious soul, intensely devoted to this experience we call life.

—Sunaina Rangnekar, multidimensional
creative and yoga guide

2

The Yamas
How You Are with Others

YOGA ETHICS WILL CHANGE your life if you practice them deeply. I know it has completely transformed mine. Yoga is a tradition that's both spiritual and exceedingly practical; it reminds us that we can't live consciously without living ethically. So, in addition to whatever values and ethics you already live by, yoga offers up the yamas and niyamas, the traditional ethical precepts of yoga. In practicing these precepts, you learn to follow your inner guidance to personal growth on emotional, physical, and spiritual levels; you commit to a life of truth, compassion, generosity, and peace. In doing so, you embark on a path of transformation, healing, and happiness for yourself, all other sentient beings, and the planet. Even if you are familiar with these precepts and practices, read them with the open eyes of a sad-haka and allow them to rekindle a spark within you. We will explore these core yogic tenets as they show up in our own lives and practices, our relationships with others, and in our work in the world.

These ethical principles aren't simply ancient words for ancient times. They are completely relevant to life right now. In fact, yoga comes alive when you bring it into your everyday life—into your challenges and your blessings, into the times you feel most creative and the times you feel bored or listless. By continuing to adapt the practice to fit into the world, practitioners keep this ever-changing form of yoga in alignment with its entire history. The key to this evolution is to ensure that teachers and practitioners are moving forward in innovative ways that remain rooted in the ancient tradition

and its foundational philosophies. In this section, we'll introduce
the eight-limbed path briefly, and then in part 2, we'll investigate
the role these practices play in our personal lives and in our commitment to compassionate service and leadership.

A sadhaka's path is to practice all the different aspects of yoga. In
any one path, you will go deeper into all.

THE YAMAS AND THE NIYAMAS

∷

The yamas and niyamas are:
- Founded in a fundamental understanding that we are
  inherently pure, whole, and good, and that we are all
  connected to one another.
- Concrete expressions of the practice and teachings of
  yoga and the Eightfold Path, and they represent a vision
  for a global yoga practice, lifestyle, and ethic.
- The way we begin to understand our responsibility as
  yoga practitioners, teachers, mentors, and guides. They
  deepen our awareness of the sensitive nature of the
  student-teacher relationship, especially the hierarchical
  power structures that advantage the teacher.

The first limb, the yamas, focuses on how you show up in the world.
The yamas are *ahimsa*, satya, *asteya, brahmacharya*, and *aparigraha*.
These five outward-facing yogic codes can help you see how your
thoughts, words, and actions impact others. Taken together, they
teach the yoga of kindness, loving speech, deep listening, care, generosity, energy management, and nonattachment; and they offer
up ways to minimize separation and divisiveness, beginning with
ahimsa and satya.

There's a reason the yamas begin with ahimsa, a vow to do no harm through your actions, thoughts, and words and to have reverence for all living beings. Ahimsa teaches that when someone's actions harm another or contribute to the destruction of the planet, they are harmed as well. Satya, or truthfulness, is next. It asks you to see things as they are, not how you would interpret them or want them to be. When we are out of integrity, separated from our soul's truth, we suffer and, in turn, we can cause suffering. Asteya is the third yama, the literal translation of which means non-stealing. I prefer to think of it as a *generosity* practice, a way of uplifting others as well as a reminder of our inherent enoughness. Brahmacharya, the fourth yama, encourages you not to squander your life force, to be mindful about how you use your energy and where you place your attention. Balance in all things! And finally, the fifth yama, aparigraha, invites you to notice what you hold on to and asks you to release what you no longer need and what fails to serve the higher good. It's important to realize that Patanjali didn't offer the yamas as "Thou Shalt Not . . ." commandments; rather, they're meant to be skillful ways to relate to the world that don't increase the world's suffering or our own.

अहिंसा AHIMSA. NONVIOLENCE OR NON-HARMING; ACTING WITH UNCONDITIONAL KINDNESS

The beautiful truth about ahimsa is it does not have to be complicated. In fact, it really is quite straightforward. It simply means being mindful of each action you do and doing it with the least harm and the most love. Ahimsa is both practical and aspirational.

In India, *ahimsakas* are those who are devoted to practicing ahimsa in every aspect of life and develop what is called "soul force"—the power that comes from practicing—that cannot be given or taken away. Being an ahimsaka, I discovered, was quite simple but not always easy. At the time, I was living and working at Maitreya, a small rural school in Bihar, where nonviolence is very much interwoven with their dedication to service. Every day we'd awaken at five in the morning to sweep ficus tree leaves from the grounds surrounding the school in the half-light. Each stroke that sweeps dust and dirt from our school grounds lays a foundation for clean, quiet minds to begin the day. After work, we'd come together as a community for morning assembly, a time for students to share stories that emphasize ethical values, practice meditation and concentration exercises, or enact scenes about conflict resolution.

Whether in the Maitreya school in rural Bihar or in a neighborhood yoga studio or in a city like London or Los Angeles, we can develop soul force by practicing ahimsa. Soul force awakens in the love we share in our classrooms, with our families, and through our actions. We harness it every time we are listening to our own hearts, attuned to the moment, acting from truth, connection, commitment, integrity, and equality. Laughing, playing, learning, we are students walking in the footsteps of those who came before us, creating our own imprints alongside the many ahimsakas of the past, present, and future.

Ahimsa is not
- being a "nice, good person"
- tone-policing folks, particularly folks of color, imploring them to show up "nicely"
- policing the way people express emotion or making them spiritually bypass
- being a vegetarian or vegan and thinking that's all that's needed to be an ahimsaka
- trying to "fix" anyone or offering your own solutions, advice, or help without being asked or invited to do so
- turning away from harm inflicted on other people

Ahimsa is
- interrupting harm wherever you find it and standing up to injustice in all its forms. A vow of nonviolence and non-harming toward yourself, others, animals, and the environment
- being kinder, compassionate, and more engaged in the world, as part of your spiritual practice that can support you

- taking a stand for healing justice, social justice, self-care, and equity
- taking *direct* action against injustice in a system that violently oppresses others, even if doing so makes you feel uncomfortable. Martin Luther King Jr. said, in his speech at Stanford University in 1967, "A riot is the language of the unheard."[1] He went on to discuss how nonviolence can create alternative ways to equity and justice. Ahimsa asks us all to listen and heed the call.

░░ AHIMSA REFLECTION QUESTIONS

Ahimsa is the first precept for a reason: it is an essential element of every yama and niyama, of everything we do in our daily lives. Sometimes it feels easier to be kind to others than it is to treat ourselves with loving respect and understanding. However, it's important that we honor ourselves, as well as our relationships and our work in the world, with true presence and loving-kindness.

For the Self
- Pay attention to how you speak to and treat your body. What are some default phrases you hear yourself repeating? How can you treat yourself kindlier?
- How might you prioritize rest and self-care?
- In your practice, what are some of the ways you can be kinder to yourself?

With Others
- In what ways do you inadvertently cause harm to those you interact with? What are some ways in which you could listen more, be kinder and more attentive?
- Pay attention to your language choices. How do they reflect your biases or jealousies and cause harm to others? How do they prevent you from having loving, meaningful, and connected relationships?

In the World

- Where might you be causing harm and what are some steps you can take to reduce it?
- As you learn and do better, how might you act?
- In what ways do your language choices; old narratives or presuppositions from your parents, grandparents, and others; and biases get in your way of listening to and learning from others and being able to contribute to the well-being of others?

⣿ Ahimsa Practice

Bring your mind, body, and heart together as you join your hands at the center of your chest in Anjali mudra. Take three deep breaths and say the following prayer, either aloud or to yourself:

> May I continue to cultivate openness and nondiscrimination toward myself and others.
> May I be nonviolent toward myself, having regard for all beings in order to practice peace and transform suffering in myself and in the world.
> May I continue to find more ways and opportunities to be kinder to myself, to the people I love, to those who cross my path, and to those I struggle to understand and appreciate.
> May I transform suffering in myself and in the world
> May I cultivate power that no one can give and no one can take away, the power of ahimsa.

Consider this yama as a reflective lake to look at yourself. Internally, say yes in your mind and heart each time you know that you have aimed to embody, live, and practice this yama.   ⣿

सत्य SATYA. TRUTHFULNESS

Satya, often translated as "telling the truth," is actually more nuanced than that. The word *sat* means "that which exists," "true essence," or "beingness." In other words, satya is the unvarnished truth, the soul's truth; it asks you to see things as they really are, not how you interpret them or would like them to be.

Practicing satya certainly means to stop telling lies or even fudging the truth—*and* it's much more than that. *Satyagraha* means "truth force" (*satya*, "truth"; *graha*, "force"). It was this force, the force of truth, that liberated India from its oppressors. It requires all of us to look within ourselves and commit to the truth of who we are without distortion. It's hard to do that when you don't *know* who you are—and even harder to model that for others. Satya also asks you to *listen deeply*, again, without the distortion of your preconceived prejudices or judgments; and to listen by engaging *all* your sense organs. The natural world communicates without words and people often do too; we can listen with not only our ears but our eyes, our heart, our touch, our speech, and all the ways we can hear another's truth into being. As Mahatma Gandhi, the nonviolent spiritual leader of the movement for Indian Independence from the British, once wrote, "There should be truth in thought, truth in speech, and truth in Action. Ahimsa is the means, but truth is the end."[2] This is the path and the call of a yoga practitioner.

There is no way to practice satya without ahimsa; and no way to practice yoga without incorporating both ahimsa and satya. A satya practice invites you to ask this question at every turn: *Is what I'm doing or saying right now creating more connection or more division? Does it serve a greater purpose or does it do harm?* This can be your yoga unity check-in as you bring satya into your everyday life. Before I say more about what satya is, let's remember what it is not.

Satya is not
- how you personally feel about an action or event
- your interpretation of something, or how you wish it could be

- a relative truth conditioned by your own biases, reactions, or ego
- a way to seek revenge or be mean-spirited—nor is it your unsolicited opinions
- telling the truth at any cost without regard to how it will be received

Satya is
- the deep, unchanging truth (i.e., the "soul's truth") that sits underneath
- an ability to sit with and hold multiple perspectives; the paradox of multiple truths that seem contradictory all being true
- deep, thoughtful listening; being open to hearing and receiving the truth from others
- what emerges when you commit to truly listening before you offer your response
- always accompanied by ahimsa so your words are offered in kindness, at the appropriate time, and with the least amount of harm

⁑ Satya Reflection Questions

Here are some questions to consider as you reflect on how to speak the truth—and receive another's truth with loving attention and without aggression or harm. In other words, how to practice ahimsa and satya simultaneously.

For the Self
- What do you know to be true about yourself?
- What is the truth that you are here to create into being?
- Think about a time when you didn't tell the truth. What were the circumstances that led to that choice? How did it make you feel? What did you learn from that experience?

With Others

- Pick someone who you feel embodies satya. This could be a person in your life, someone you know or have heard about, a historical figure, or an activist. What are the qualities of that person that you specifically see? How do they model satya? Be as detailed and descriptive as possible.
- How do you embody those same qualities yourself? How do you model satya in your relationships, whether they're intimate or casual? Be specific.

In the World

- Think about a time when you said or did something that caused more separation than unity. How did that feel? What were the circumstances surrounding that action?
- Think about a time when you showed up in truth in your community and with those you are in service to. What helped you do that? What can you put in place to keep that happening?
- How can you explore other truths that may be different from yours but still remain committed to your own path?
- What is the essence, the truth, of your commitment to social justice?
- How can you offer your truth in service to others without ignoring or dismissing their truth?

⁚⁚ SATYA PRACTICE

Bring your mind, body, and heart together as you join your hands at the center of your chest in Anjali mudra. Take three deep breaths and say the following prayer, either aloud or to yourself:

> May I practice truthful thinking, speech, and action in order to promote growth and peace in myself and among others.
> May I listen deeply to hear others into their own truths.

May I pause before speaking and use open communication to resolve any conflicts.

May I remember that what I think, do, and say can create
happiness or suffering, so I vow to use my actions, words,
and listening to inspire joy, confidence, and positivity.

May I use my voice to speak up for social justice.

Consider this yama as a reflective lake to look at yourself. Internally,
say yes in your mind each time you know that you have aimed to
embody, live, and practice this yama.   ⁑

अस्तेय ASTEYA. NON-STEALING AND GENEROSITY

On the surface, asteya is pretty straightforward. It asks you not to
take what doesn't belong to you, not to covet what other people
have, and not to use more than your share of resources. It's easy to
see how this applies to other people's *stuff*. It can also apply when
you feel insecure, unfulfilled, or "less than" and attempt to fill that
void by stealing other people's attention, affection, ideas, energy, or
strength so you can feel better about yourself.

By practicing asteya, you can begin to experience a sense of inner
abundance, which gives rise to knowing that you have everything
you need within you. You *are* enough. It doesn't deny your challenges or your "failures." Instead, it asks you to freely acknowledge
the whole of yourself, to say yes to life, and to remember to be tender
and forgiving with yourself. Asteya awakens within you the realization that *being* enough does not imply that everyone *has* enough—
food, shelter, emotional support, or adequate transportation. It
becomes a practice of generosity—of giving up and giving back.

When you embrace this sense of *enoughness*, you no longer feel
the need to take more than your share of the resources that belong
(or should belong) to everyone; your practice can now include
working toward and supporting the personal, systemic, and political
changes necessary to enable others to also have enough; you're able
to give more freely to others from the abundance you enjoy and let
go of the need to appropriate what is not yours to take.

Asteya is a powerful teaching for those of us living in capitalism or really any system that places worth on how much we can produce, extract, and consume. It is directly related to the human condition of craving for more to fill a sense of lack. Instead of stealing from ourselves, our time, our experiences, and our lives, it challenges us to pause, to see that we already have enough, despite all the messaging of lack we are bombarded with in advertisements and social media posts; and from our families, schools, and communities, as well as the culture in which we live. Think of asteya as an abundance practice that can bring about a shift in perspective from "What am I missing?" to "What can I appreciate?" From "What am I appropriating" to "What can I uplift?"

Asteya is not
- accumulating material wealth and power
- looking to others for validation of your worth
- practicing selective generosity—giving to some and not others
- holding back—giving a little but withholding as well
- only personal—you can also be stealing others' opportunities by systemic advantage

Asteya is
- becoming conscious of what keeps you stuck
- freely acknowledging the "all of you"—your challenges, "faults," or "failures"—saying yes to life, and remembering to be tender and forgiving with yourself
- a gratitude practice—remembering that you don't need to appropriate anything from anyone else; you have enough, you *are* enough
- returning what doesn't belong to you
- lifting up others by supporting and honoring their work
- shifting perspective from "What am I missing?" to "What can I appreciate?"

⁞⁞ Asteya Reflection Questions

It's important to consider how practicing asteya can help minimize any harm you do to yourself and others and how it can help you show up fully in the world.

For the Self
- Think of a time you allowed your own voice to drown out the voice of another.
- Consciously remind yourself that you *are* enough, you matter, and your contribution is important.
- Identify and reflect on times when you feel out of integrity with who you really are.
- Identify and reflect on your own power. How might you apply asteya personally and culturally?

With Others
- What do you allow others to take from you? What have you appropriated from others?
- What are some ways you can show gratitude to those who have taught you well? Some ways you give them credit for what you've learned?
- Think of ways in which you've been able to practice the compassionate trifecta of ahimsa, satya, and asteya—toward yourself and others.

In the World
- What kinds of actions can you take to create a world that sees and acknowledges your and other people's strengths and assets rather than focusing on lack?
- Often the alternative to appropriation is creativity. Where can you tune in to your own culture, background, and experiences and build from there?

⁚⁚ ASTEYA PRACTICE

Bring your mind, body, and heart together as you join your hands at the center of your chest in Anjali mudra. Take three deep breaths and say the following prayer, either aloud or to yourself:

> May I honor what belongs to others and celebrate what has been given to me.
> May I live from abundance, remembering I have everything I need right here, inside of myself.
> May I cultivate a deep satisfaction with life.
> May I be mindful of my consumption and not consume from a sense of lack or fear.
> May I consume in ways that allow for others to also have what they need.
> May I stand against oppressive systems that exploit and create more justice and equity for all.
> May I practice coming back to the present moment; to be in the presence of the miracles all around me and to connect with all that is.

Consider this yama as a reflective lake to look at yourself. Internally, say yes in your mind each time you know that you have aimed to embody, live, and practice this yama. ⁚⁚

ब्रह्मचर्य BRAHMACHARYA. ALIGNED USE OF ENERGY OR CONSTANCY

Brahmacharya can be translated as "following the path of Brahma," the "middle path of restraint," or more poetically "walking in the presence of the divine." Brahmacharya encourages you to channel your energy, your life force, toward a higher or more spiritual purpose. It invites you to direct your attention inward in order to control and balance the senses; to pledge constancy or fidelity to the teachings and a more conscious, values-based life. Practicing brahmacharya can help you be mindful and deliberate about how you use and direct your energy so you can experience a sense of contentment and peace. It can help you set boundaries and better manage your energy so you can stay focused on your divine purpose.

Back in Vedic times, brahmacharya was the first of the four stages of life, or ashramas—the stage of the student, a time of learning. Students promised that they would conserve and focus all their energy—life force, breath, and sexual energy—on gaining knowledge through education. The ancients believed that the energy that stimulates our sexual pleasures is the same energy that propels our spiritual pursuits. So they felt it was important not to squander it in our youth on more puerile interests. As such, brahmacharya has come to be associated with celibacy, which is great if you're an aspiring monk; not so great if you're a householder, a person concerned with worldly pursuits. Householder is one of the traditional Vedic life stages: student, householder, forest dweller, renunciate. A householder is someone connected to worldly, not just spiritual, pursuits.

Before we look at what it means to practice brahmacharya as a householder, let's get clear on what it is and what it is not.

Brahmacharya is not
- only a vow of celibacy
- a practice of self-sacrifice or denial
- doing only what you want, whenever you want
- unquestioning obedience to a guru
- giving away your power and agency

Brahmacharya is
- a focused commitment to self-care and community care
- taking to heart the depth of learning as a student of yoga
- an invitation to channel your energy and not squander it
- a devotion practice
- a practice to learn lessons and direct your senses
- a natural dance of giving and receiving
- Permission to check in with yourself, create and hold boundaries

⠿ Brahmacharya Reflection Questions

Practicing brahmacharya helps us know ourselves on an intimate level so that we can be in relationship with and of service out in the world with constancy and commitment, in alignment with our truth. Consider the following questions.

For the Self

- How do the actions or demands of another align with your principles? Do they take you away from your commitments or bring you closer to your purpose?
- What does your body need from you and how can you best manage your self-care?
- How can you set boundaries for your own well-being and still honor your relationships?
- What can you commit to in your daily, weekly, or monthly practice with regularity? What do you have to give up—or add in—in order to center your sadhana practice?

With Others

- Which relationships increase your energy and which ones drain it?
- How can you give energy to relationships and actions that nourish and support you and let go of negative attachments that do harm?
- Where are the energy leaks in your life—social media, endless to-do lists, obligations that no longer serve you, one-sided relationships, toxic family dynamics? How can you plug those leaks?
- What do you need to do to take care of yourself within relationships in order to protect your soul-force energy?

In the World

- What feels important to spend your energy on?
- What does the world need from you and how can you best serve?

- Ask yourself, "Am I serving others to gratify my need for recognition or because I want to support others' growth and development?"
- What gets in your way of directing your energy toward the highest good—for yourself and for others?

⁘ BRAHMACHARYA PRACTICE

Bring your mind, body, and heart together as you join your hands at the center of your chest in Anjali mudra. Take three deep breaths, in and out, and say the following prayer, either aloud or to yourself:

> Knowing my energy is sacred, may I respect and cherish it.
> May I respect and honor the boundaries of others, ask for and honor consent.
> May I connect to the universal abundant replenishment of energy in spiritual sources.
> May I direct my energy to preserve positive and uplifting experiences for myself and others.
> May I do my best to cultivate love, kindness, compassion, joy, and inclusiveness as the elements of true love and care.
> May I continue to practice devotion to the divine.

Listen with an open mind and heart. Consider this yama as a reflective lake to look at yourself. Internally, say yes in your mind each time you know that you have aimed to embody, live, and practice this yama.   ⁘

अपरिग्रह APARIGRAHA. THE POWER OF LETTING GO

Aparigraha is freedom from constraints such as attachment, greed, or desire that can get in the way of you living the purposeful life you are meant to live. Aparigraha allows you to let go of anything that prevents you from stepping deeper into your own truth and allowing others to do the same. Broken down etymologically, *a*, means "not," *pari* means "all sides" or "in all ways," and *graha* means "to grab, seek, or crave." Together, *aparigraha* means not taking more than you need or coveting what you don't have; it is practicing nonaccumulation; and it is letting go of your attachment to what you have (or what you covet). All of this can lead to independence, trust, and self-sovereignty. As the *Ashtavakra Gita* says, "Your desires are your downfall. When you want nothing, you need nothing. When you need nothing, all the universe is yours."[3] Aparigraha is one of the foundational tenets of yoga and, for me, a big invitation to go deeper into personal practice.

Aparigraha, of course, applies to more than tangible things or physical objects. It also asks you to examine your thoughts and biases, even your relationships, to see which ones contribute to your suffering and the suffering of others—and commit to releasing their hold on you. Deepening in aparigraha can remind you that everything has a beginning, middle, and end; that there is a depth you can come to by letting go of attachment, by simplifying your life. There's a way that holding on to things can hold you back from being who you are meant to be—and offering the gifts you are meant to offer.

I think it's important to distinguish between *having* things and being possessed or defined by them. For example, you may need to buy a car. You find one that you really like and it has everything you want. You may even get a lot of pleasure out of driving it. If, however, you begin to measure your self-worth by the coolness of your new purchase—and can't imagine life without it—your happiness becomes dependent on an *external* source of pleasure. You have, as the Indian teacher and yoga pioneer B. K. S. Iyengar said, "an addiction to the furniture of life, instead of . . . the joy of life."[4]

So often I find myself fluctuating between craving something or running away from it. Practicing aparigraha provides a sacred pause—a moment of stillness in between desiring something and acting on that desire. That is where you can drop into that space of freedom in the practice of aparigraha.

Aparigraha is not

- having to give up all your relationships and possessions and live a monk's life
- the belief you cannot take pleasure in external things or relationships
- a way to make you feel ashamed, fearful, or a victim

Aparigraha is

- a way to release your attachment to a certain image of yourself and make space for something new to grow
- a practice of gratitude
- a reminder not to hold on too tightly to relationships or look to others for your happiness
- a practice of getting "unstuck" from desire and opening to what really matters

⁘ Aparigraha Reflection Questions

Aparigraha opens our hearts beyond our own desires and reminds us that we are enough just as we are, that we can paradoxically experience abundance by ridding ourselves of possessions, ideas, and relationships that we no longer need. Here are some questions to consider:

For the Self

- What do you hold on to long past its expiration date? It could be boxes of memories you've carted around with you for years, a place you know in your heart of hearts doesn't feel like home anymore, or maybe a closet full of clothes that no longer work for you.
- What was the hardest possession to give away? The easiest? Were you surprised?
- Who are you without your possessions? Is it possible to loosen the grip around what you cling to or how you define yourself?
- Can you find a pause between your craving and aversion?

With Others
- What can you let go of right now? What have you outgrown?
- Is there any part of your relationships (with your partner, children, and friends, or at work) that needs more spaciousness, understanding, and trust? What do you need to let go of to make that happen?
- How can aparigraha help you make better choices in your relationships? Are there people or connections you are ready to let go of? Others you'd like to get to know but you've had no room for?
- If you are attached to doing things a certain way, see if you can loosen your grip a little bit and try something new instead. How did that feel?

In the World
- Who are you underneath your attachments?
- Are you willing to let go of what gets in your way of listening to other points of view?
- Have you ever had to give up your own comforts to stand up for what is right and to serve the greater good? What was that like?
- What are the biases, old stories, or values you were taught as a child that are getting in the way of you showing up fully for justice? What can you replace them with?

⠿ APARIGRAHA PRACTICE

Bring your mind, body, and heart together as you join your hands at the center of your chest in Anjali mudra. Take three deep breaths, in and out.

May all beings be free from attachment and aversion.
May I let go of expectations.
May I remember that impermanence is part of life, that change is constant.

May I find freedom in surrendering what no longer serves
me or the greater good.
May I be committed to cultivating the insight of interbeing
and compassion.

Listen with an open mind and heart. Consider this yama as a reflective lake to look at yourself. Internally, say yes in your mind each
time you know that you have aimed to embody, live, and practice
this yama.   ::

3

The Niyamas
How You Care for Your Spiritual Self

THE NIYAMAS—inward-facing ethical codes—can guide you toward a deeper understanding of yourself. They go beyond the external into your internal landscape, asking the question: *How can these practices minimize the suffering within me, help me live more closely aligned to my divine nature, and lead me toward true liberation?*

The niyamas begin with *saucha*, cleanliness or purity, an invitation to simplify your life, by removing the physical, mental, and emotional obstacles that get in the way of living with presence, integrity, and purpose. Next is *santosha*, the practice of being content and peaceful, finding pockets of happiness no matter what you're faced with and knowing that you have within you the capacity for pure joy. The third niyama, *tapas*—meaning "self-discipline," "heat," or "willpower"—helps you burn away anything that clouds your true nature and reclaim your sense of purpose and inner joy. *Svadhyaya* invites you to know yourself more deeply through self-reflection and self-study. It can be a tool to increase self-confidence and banish negative self-talk, reminding you of the gifts you have to share with others. And finally you open to contemplate the universe, spiritual truths, and take your very own seat of being with *ishvara pranidhana*.

शौच SAUCHA. CLEANLINESS, PURITY, CLARITY

Saucha literally means "purity or cleanliness." It applies to not only how you treat your physical body and your surroundings but also how you work with your thoughts and emotions and the not-so-skillful habits that have a hold on you. It helps to think about saucha as akin to ahimsa—that is, as an invitation to be mindful of your actions, to show up with a pure heart, and to be conscious of the ways in which you fail to do so. Saucha also connects back to aparigraha, encouraging you to let go of the clutter in your life (and in your mind) that prevents you from finding the clarity you need to direct your attention—and your actions—toward the greater good.

Saucha invites all of us to be in respectful relationship with our surroundings and our belongings. That, of course, includes our practice spaces and what we choose to put in them. I truly believe the more serene you can make your space, the more spacious and comfortable you'll feel. This is true even when your space is tiny. It isn't just about decluttering your physical space, however. It's also about caring for and honoring your body. It means treating your body with tenderness and respect, being mindful of how you nourish yourself, and practicing self-love; committing to a physical practice that feels appropriate at any given moment. It is also a way of cleansing your mind of anything that blocks or distracts you from being truly present. It can help you be more mindful of how your thoughts, words, and actions can negatively (or positively) impact your relationships or your work in the world. When your mind is clear, when you can direct your energy toward being more receptive, it's easier to welcome new experiences and be open to groups of people you may have previously shut out because of limiting beliefs or fears. Practicing saucha gives you a clearer sense of what your gifts are and how you might serve others.

Saucha is not
- simply cleaning your space and thinking you are done with this practice
- feeling like you need to go directly from impure to pure
- a way of making you feel bad about yourself and your actions

Saucha is
- a practice of connecting the internal and external for liberation

- living with simple wisdom as a guide
- loving yourself as you clear out what is unsupportive of growth
- entering into relationship with your external spaces as well as your internal landscape

⁝⁝ SAUCHA REFLECTION QUESTIONS

Saucha invites us to reflect on where we are in alignment with our true self and highest intentions. To clear out that which gets in the way so nothing separates us and the divine.

Here are some questions to consider:

For the Self

- What thoughts can you clear away that are taking up too much space in your mind?
- How might you set up your practice space so that it feels sacred?
- What are some ways you can practice simplicity?

With Others

- How can you clear away distractions so you show up fully present for someone in your life?
- How do your thoughts, words, and actions negatively (or positively) impact your relationships or your work in the world?
- Where and how can you get to the simplest way of connecting with another being?

In the World

- What do you wish you could clear away on a cultural or systemic level? Tapping into the wish "to clear away" that drives your action in the world is powerful.
- How can you practice, be more receptive, and welcome new experiences; be open to other cultures, groups of people, or even new foods and practices?
- What are some ways you'd like your practice of saucha to

give you a clearer sense of what your gifts are and how you might serve others?

❖ SAUCHA PRACTICE

Bring your mind, body, and heart together as you join your hands at the center of your chest in Anjali mudra. Take three deep breaths, in and out.

> May I listen with an open mind and heart.
> May I keep my mind, body, and surroundings clean and pure and treat them with loving respect.
> May I honor my living space by maintaining a clean and well-organized household.
> May I treat my body with loving respect.
> May I practice right speech and right action so that my words and efforts do no harm.
> May I create space and time for purification and clearing out what no longer serves the highest good.

Consider this niyama as a beautiful pool of clear water to look deeply in at ourselves. Internally, say yes in your mind each time you know that you have aimed to embody, live, and practice this niyama.   ❖

संतोष SANTOSHA. CONTENTMENT, SATISFACTION

When I think of santosha, I think about the pure, unadulterated joy that comes when I'm fully alive in the moment. *Santosha* means "completely content," or as B. K. S. Iyengar describes, when "the rhythm of the body, the melody of the mind, and the harmony of the soul [come together to] create the symphony of life."[1] Santosha invites you to explore for yourself what truly brings you joy and contentment—not what your friends, family, or society think *should* bring you joy or contentment but what you know to be true.

Santosha is not synonymous with pleasure; it's also not about chasing after what you *think* or hope will make you happy. If you just get that job, find the perfect relationship, get the attention you crave, you'll be content. It doesn't work that way! All of your "if onlys" and "as soon as" just get in the way of remembering that you *already* have everything you need to be content. In fact, joy resides within each of us.

Yoga teaches that suffering also arises from chasing after and holding on to pleasure while doing whatever you can to push pain away. It's not that pleasure is a bad thing; it's that often your attachment to it can ironically make you more miserable. In practicing santosha, you begin to understand that pain and pleasure are the same, that you can welcome both pleasure *and* pain without being ruled by either one. You can feel everything as it arises without holding on to expectations.

Santosha asks you to plant yourself firmly in the present moment, noticing and being content with what is happening *as it's happening*. It's helpful to think of santosha as a practice of "being with"—a practice that invites you to stay present to whatever arises. Feel everything. When you're angry, let yourself be angry. If you are full of joy and pleasure, feel that. It's about equanimity—*upekkha* in Pali—which means standing in the middle, seeing without getting caught by what you're seeing. As one of my teachers used to ask, What was your face before you were born? What are you here to experience and create?

Santosha is not
- chasing after what you think will make you happy
- holding on to what makes you happy and pushing away what makes you unhappy
- synonymous with pleasure
- dependent on other people's thoughts and actions
- complacency or self-sacrifice; it's not settling for less than you deserve

Santosha is
- finding clarity and peace within yourself
- noticing and being content with what is happening as it's happening
- taking delight in the everyday moments that life brings your way
- a way of immersing yourself in the here and now until time slips away
- the gateway to more clarity, ease, and well-being

▪▪ Santosha Reflection Questions

Joy comes when we begin to uncover the truths that allow us to be more in alignment with who we are; when we can be absolutely sovereign with what brings us contentment and joy. There are many ways to access the practice of santosha. Here are some questions to consider:

For the Self
- What brings you joy and contentment? Not what your friends, family, or society thinks should bring you joy or make you content but what truly brings you joy and ease.
- Think back to your childhood. Leaving aside challenging or hard moments in this visualization, what were some moments of pure delight?
- What are some of the things you do that cause you to lose a sense of time and space? For some of us, this might be art, cooking, painting, meditation, running, dancing, or other forms of joyful practice.

With Others
- What are some of the things that bring collective joy to your relationships?
- What stands in your way of being fully present to others? What do you need to set aside in order to prioritize the here and now?

- What do you truly appreciate about your relationships?
- In your family, how can you create a warm and connected environment in which each person can be their highest and best self?

In the World

- How can a commitment to santosha uplift your community as a whole as well as those who benefit from the work you do?
- How would you like your practice of santosha to contribute to the creative work of your community?
- What are practices that can be put in place to sow the seeds of contentment and minimize the opportunities for discontent or frustration?
- What stands in your way of participating or committing fully?
- What are the "spirit children" you are creating together? For example, if you are part of a group of yoga teachers, how can you work toward creating a space for more deep and authentic practice? If you are organizers and activists, how can you cocreate artwork and movements for liberation?

░ Santosha Practice

Bring your mind, body, and heart together as you join your hands at the center of your chest in Anjali mudra. Take three deep breaths, in and out. Listen with an open mind and heart.

May I cultivate joy in as many moments as possible.
May I turn my mind toward gratitude to nourish my contentment.
May I vow to grow and learn from the events in my life.
May I strive to have a positive outlook, learn from others, and work toward peace.
May I let grace and faith guide all events and fill every activity.

May I take pleasure in the present moment, doing what I love and enjoying myself.
May I bring care and uplift to all the beings I encounter.

Consider this niyama as a beautiful pool of clear water in which to look deeply within. Internally, say yes in your mind each time you know that you have aimed to embody, live, and practice this niyama.   ⁑

तपस् TAPAS: SPIRITUAL WILLPOWER

Tapas comes from the Sanskrit root *tap*, which means "to burn." Tapas is the internal flame that motivates you and is closely associated with *agni*, the fire element or incarnation of fire in the *Rig Veda* and other Vedic texts. Tapas is more than just the third niyama, however; it is an essential part of Kriya Yoga, Patanjali's schematic action plan, along with *svadhyaya* and *ishvara pranidhana*, that brings yoga into your everyday life through discipline, self-understanding, and humility.

The many translations of tapas—"fire"; "heat"; "discipline, dedication, and determination"; "willpower"; "austerity"; and "simplicity"— all point to one thing: singleness of purpose; a willingness to burn away everything that blocks your ability to truly know who you are. Simplify, focus, keep showing up with full attention. Shed old habits or patterns of behavior that get in the way of your spiritual growth. Tapas is the fire that allows you to create the space you need for true transformation to happen. Sometimes that means doing a little emotional housecleaning and saying goodbye to old relationships that have run their course. Tapas intensifies your desire to commit to and work with all the yamas and niyamas more deeply.

You may make many choices and actions that are in alignment with your true essence, that band of unwavering light within. And you no doubt may make many choices that lead you away from that aligned center. Ten, fifteen, a hundred choices off track. It doesn't matter. When that happens, tapas arises as a form of *abhyasa*—that is, a regular, consistent, and mindful practice. It keeps you coming back, coming back, coming back without judgment or scolding. Yoga is such a beautiful and supportive practice.

Tapas is not

- being overly committed to the point of exhaustion or burn-out—in other words, burning the candle at both ends
- pushing yourself harder than your physical, mental, or emotional energy can handle
- acting from fear of not being "enough" or not working hard enough
- an excuse to act out of anger, agitation, or impatience

Tapas is

- the discipline you need to get up in the morning and get moving
- stepping out of your comfort zone
- the commitment to do the work you are here to do and to stay the course
- stoking your self-confidence, drive, and willpower to keep going
- the practice of emotional or internal housecleaning and building spiritual willpower

:: TAPAS REFLECTION QUESTIONS

Tapas is a dance of ritual and discipline. It's setting your alarm at 5:00 a.m. for a sunrise sadhana. It's gathering sacred objects, water, fire, ghee, flowers, around the *murthi*, or altar, for ritual. All these devotion, discipline, and ritual practices build heat and spiritual fire for deep practice. It is listening to what your body needs, sometimes diving deeper into your physical practice; other times prioritizing rest, meditation, walks in nature, or play. Some questions to consider:

For the Self

- What ignites your spiritual willpower for practice?
- What are you ready to let go of, to burn up, that no longer works for you? What do you want to make room for?
- Is there anything that gets in your way of having a consistent sadhana practice? Or of having a friendlier relationship with your body or your mind?
- How can you use tapas to motivate you to create new habits? To let go of negative self-talk and embrace your "enoughness" and your inner strength?

With Others

- What can you "burn up" that gets in your way of prioritizing and being truly present in your primary relationships?
- Are there relationships in your life—at home, at work, within your circle of friends or community—that have gone on too long and that you can let go of or give less attention to?
- How can tapas on the mat help you create a practice that works for you at that moment?

In the World

- How can you use tapas as a practice of holding "useful" tension in your community, which can be a bridge to taking action?
- What is calling to you on a cultural or systemic level? What drives your passion?
- What is yoga asking of you right now? How can you heed the call? What gets in your way of saying yes?
- How can you ignite the fire within you to support the (r)evolution you are building?

⁘ TAPAS PRACTICE

Bring your mind, body, and heart together as you join your hands at the center of your chest in Anjali mudra. Take three deep breaths, in and out. Listen with an open mind and heart.

May I commit to my practice with discipline and focus.
May I harness yogic discipline for the power of good.
May I feed the fire within to change myself for the better.
May I cultivate and find enthusiasm for daily spiritual practice.
May I apply consistent effort to maintaining wellness with a steady application of energy.
May I balance discipline and devotion.

Consider this niyama as a beautiful pool of clear water in which to look deeply within. Internally, say yes in your mind each time you know that you have aimed to embody, live, and practice this niyama.

स्वाध्याय Svadhyaya: Self-Reflection

Svadhyaya is knowing the divine through self-study or self-reflection. *Sva* (स्व) means "own," "one's own," "self," "the human soul"; *dhyaya* (ध्याय) means "meditating on." Where tapas is the willpower, determination, and focus you need to do the work, svadhyaya is how you meet, witness, and engage with the work in order to understand the shadow parts of yourself that keep you separate. Many find reading sacred texts, modern spiritual books, or poetry can move them into that contemplative space of self-inquiry with patience and curiosity.

A deep emptiness arises when you forget how to connect with yourself, leading to confusion, a sense of loss, emptiness, and a lack of direction. Svadhyaya provides an embodied path of self-remembering. I also think of svadhyaya as resting in awareness. We are divine, universal consciousness and this practice helps us remember, explore, and get to know ourselves in a much deeper, more interconnected way.

Svadhyaya can also help you not get so focused on tapas that you burn out. It can be that self-calibrating check-in. Where tapas provides the willpower to practice harder—even when you don't feel like it—svadhyaya provides the pause in which the inquiry becomes:

How am I doing? What do I need right now? There is so much wisdom in this pause.

Svadhyaya can also be practiced socially. Practicing svadhyaya collectively helps you look at your positionality, power, and privilege. By exploring where you truthfully hold privilege and power, you can begin to more fully understand and practice ahimsa and truthfulness.

Svadhyaya is not
- self-absorption or self-conceit
- an act of comparison or judgment
- dependent on or the same as someone else's path or wisdom

Svadhyaya is
- the act of getting to know yourself
- the pause between thought and action
- nonjudgmental self-awareness
- being gentle and truthful in your self-inquiry (internal ahimsa and satya practice)

⁘ Svadhyaya Reflection Questions

Svadhyaya can help you explore where you are purposeful and meaningful in your life and your work for justice. It can inspire you to follow your own path, to explore your spiritual and personal journey with yoga roots and share skills for human uplift. Svadhyaya ultimately turns you back toward your inner teacher and ignites what is already within you. Here are a few questions to ponder:

For the Self
- Who are you when nobody's watching or listening?
- What does your body want you to know right now?
- Where are you in alignment with your purpose and where do you veer from that?
- What books, teachers, or practices have deepened your connection to the self?

With Others

- How has your self-inquiry impacted how you get along with others, especially those you struggle with?
- What gets in your way of connecting with others?
- How might svadhyaya deepen your practice of the yamas?

In the World

- Consider the many ways you hold power and privilege. How does your positionality impact your ability to serve?
- What legacy are you trying to build? And how can practicing self-inquiry help you do that?
- What do you have to let go of in order to show up for others in love and truth?

◦◦ Svadhyaya Practice

Slow down to be present and to practice the truth of yourself, of interconnectedness. Within yourself you find this interconnected whole. Bring your mind, body, and heart together as you join your hands at the center of your chest in Anjali mudra. Take three deep breaths, in and out. Listen with an open mind and heart.

> Through understanding myself may I come to understand all.
> May I commit to studying myself and may I trust what my body is telling me right now.
> May I know my purpose now, this year, this lifetime.
> May I observe my actions and inquire within with curiosity and nonjudgment.
> May I stay attentive to what needs to be let go and what needs care and nourishment.
> May I support another's self-knowledge.
> May I practice self-rule and stand for my own sovereignty.
> May I support others' experiences of sovereignty in the world now.

Consider this niyama as a beautiful pool of clear water in which to look deeply within. Internally, say yes in your mind each time you know that you have aimed to embody, live, and practice this niyama.

ईश्वर प्रणिधान Ishvara Pranidhana: The Power of Surrender

Ishvara pranidhana means to surrender to the divine; to offer up the fruits of your actions without being attached to a particular outcome or a particular method. It means dedicating the merits you've accumulated—through consistent practice or because of your privilege or social location—to something bigger than yourself so that your practice can, in some small way, benefit all beings. Ishvara pranidhana is a call to move *beyond* the ego, beyond the selfishness of your "small" self, and create more space to connect with the *selflessness* of your highest self. It is a radical truth underneath (and untouched by) the ego's desires.

Ishvara translates as "Supreme Being," "Universe," "Absolute Reality," your "true self," or "personal god or goddess"—in essence, something greater than yourself. *Pranidhana* means "complete surrender," "complete recognition," or "at the center of life." In surrendering to the mystery, you open to a deeper connection to all beings. In shedding the ego in favor of opening to the divine, you begin to see that there is no separation between you and other beings. And that it is your duty, your dharma—to give back to humanity what you have received through your inner work. Actively offer loving and compassionate service in ways that alleviate the suffering caused by racism, ageism, ableism, homophobia, transphobia, fatphobia (and the many cultural and systemic inequities). As the Sanskrit scholar and spiritual head of the Himalayan Institute Pandit Rajmani Tigunait says, we must then invest "our personal achievement in the general welfare of all living beings. All the world's great traditions talk of inner purification, and every form of inner purification involves an active practice of love and compassion, giving and sharing."[2]

Ishvara pranidhana is also sovereignty within the present moment and within oneself. This self-rule arises through deep practice and critical thinking. There is an inner power that yoga brings that no one else can touch. No one can give us this power and no one can take it away. It's like a dance or surrender and includes a dance of self-knowledge to the divine knower in each of us.

Ishvara pranidhana is not
- blind obedience or surrender to an outside deity
- a sign of weakness or giving up
- adherence to a particular religion, deity, or dogma
- the same for everyone
- an easy practice to let go of your limiting beliefs

Ishvara pranidhana is
- giving up your need to control and not being attached to the outcome
- a call to selfless service; offering up the fruits of your practice and your actions to the greater good
- letting go of the fragments of your "small" self and creating space for your higher self
- devotion and connection to the divine light within
- a conscious practice that allows your capacity for limitless, unconditional love to shine forth
- a way to deepen in spirit, to enliven and enrich your personal sadhana

⁙ Ishvara Pranidhana Reflections

The practice of ishvara pranidhana is the ultimate surrender to faith and trust. I love to think of it as dancing in devotion to the divine within. It is through this connection to our divine essence that we begin to understand our dharma is to serve others, not because we insist on a particular outcome but because we understand the interconnectedness of all beings. Sheena Sood, a yoga teacher and social justice advocate, reminded me that there is an ancient Sanskrit proverb, *vasudhaiva kutumbakam*, which means "the world is one family."

We all share the same ancestral origins and connection to Source, she says, and to integrate yoga and social justice is to commit oneself to a holistic state of collective liberation for our global family.[3]

For the Self
- What beliefs, practices, or fears get in your way of giving up the desire to control an outcome?
- Spend time each day in this devotion and practice. As you come out, consider writing in a journal or jotting down a few notes. What did you feel most connected to?
- Make time for contemplative practices, such as yoga nidra, to guide you into stillness

With Others
- Consider how the practice of surrendering to spirit can bring a sense of calm or openness to your relationships.
- Consider offering up to others the fruits of any action or practice that could be of benefit to them.
- Notice what it feels like to see the divine in another person. How does that change how you feel about them? How does it change the dynamic of your interactions?

In the World
- Remembering that ishvara pranidhana leads to selfless service, what does your surrender practice open you up to?
- As you let go of the need to be right, to be indispensable, how does that impact your ability to serve others? To fight for social justice?

❖ Ishvara Pranidhana Practice

Bring your mind, body, and heart together as you join your hands at the center of your chest in Anjali mudra. Take three deep breaths, in and out. Listen with an open mind and heart.

May I live yoga and may yoga live through me—today and all days.

May I be aware of the interconnection of all beings and honor energies greater than myself.

May my devotion to the divine strengthen my relationships and my work with others.

May I experience life as meaningful.

May I continue to be devoted to higher purpose, in service to spirit, and live a good life for myself and others.

May I remember that in connecting to one, I am connected to all.

Consider this niyama as a beautiful pool of clear water in which to look deeply within. Internally, say yes in your mind each time you know that you have aimed to embody, live, and practice this niyama.

The yamas and niyamas are a beautiful way to connect with the essence of yoga. They provide a language, a context in which it's possible to speak and experience yoga directly—as if it were a good friend. They guide us to find moments of stillness amid the busyness of our daily lives to unfold the wisdom within the teachings. And they prepare us to explore the eight limbs of yoga, which moves us deeper toward liberation—for ourselves and all other beings.

4

Asana, Pranayama, and Pratyahara

Vessels for Voyage

A PARABLE IN INDIA tells the story of a respected yogi who likened the Eightfold Path of yoga to preparing a vessel for a sacred voyage: The body and mind are the vessel, and these practices are the preparation for your journey inward. This preparation is not just about physical strength or flexibility; it's about cultivating an ethical, disciplined life that aligns with the deepest truths of our existence.

The yogic journey unfolds in two beautifully intertwined pathways: the external (*bahiranga*) and the internal (*antaranga*). The external path, which can feel like taking the first few steps into a mystical forest, is made up of four practices: the yamas (the compass of social ethics) and niyamas (the map of personal virtues), which we spoke about in the previous chapters; asana (the dance of physical postures), and pranayama (the rhythm of breath control).

The internal path is the heart of the journey, consisting of dharana (focused concentration), dhyana (meditative absorption), and samadhi (union with the divine). It's here, in the quiet depths of our being, that the true transformation occurs. Pratyahara is the bridge between the outer and inner worlds, inviting us into a realm where senses are harnessed and attention is turned inward, paving the way for antaranga. The journey through the inner and outer worlds is not a linear progression but rather a spiral, where external practices deepen our internal experience, and our inner growth enriches our engagement with the world. Each step, each practice, builds on the last, leading us closer to a profound spiritual awakening.

The practice of yoga is not just a path but a dance between the external and internal, each step a note in the symphony of spiritual growth. In this dance we find not just flexibility and peace but a deep connection to the essence of who we are.

ASANA: THE SEAT OF PRACTICE

Asana, one limb of the Eightfold Path, needs little introduction. Many who practice yoga today do some sort of physical postures—or are familiar with them. After all, there's incredible power in asana, the physical practice of yoga, which is part of why it's so popular worldwide. We are embodied beings. Our bodies appreciate the time to move, stretch, and strengthen, as well as the opportunity to settle, to slow down, to unify with the breath and everything else in the universe. Asana supports us in mindfulness on and off our mat.

As vital as asana is, it's not the whole yoga story! When yoga came to the West, it moved from the East Coast and eventually toward the West Coast following the Hindu spiritual leader and philosopher Swami Vivekananda's 1893 address at the World's Parliament of Religions in Chicago.[1] Many who were involved in Hollywood and show business began to flock to his teaching discourses. This meeting of spiritual philosophy and physical culture became a perfect combination for the physical practices to rise to the foreground. However, asana was never meant to stand on its own; yoga was never about focusing solely on the physical body for its own sake. In the Yoga Sutras, asana is a noun, a thing. It's the seat you take to prepare for and to sit in meditation. Patanjali says you choose that seat deliberately—what you sit on, where you sit, and how you sit. Patanjali's only requirement is that your seat be balanced between steadiness (*sthira*) and ease (*sukha*). You should feel planted and comfortable. Not too tight, not too loose. When we achieve that (even for a few breaths), our practice guides us into present-moment inquiry. We experience that steadiness and a certain sweetness, groundedness and comfort in our own container—not just our physical container but a steadiness and ease within our energy body, our mental body, our wisdom body, and our bliss body. Once that happens—it's not always easy to do—we are then invited to move into stillness and listen to what arises from within.

What emerges are the stories of your lived wisdom expressed through your body—hidden within the tissues, the bone marrow, and in every cell of the body. Every person has their unique stories; every person expresses and lives those stories in their own way. As we bend and stretch, strengthen and release, asana allows us to bring to light those stories that our body holds and desires to tell. Sometimes those stories are ancient, bequeathed to us by our ancestors; other times they are the residue from our own past experiences or questions we're trying to work through. Asana gives us a script, a language the body understands; a way of relating to the parts of our inner landscape we rarely visit. Other times it invites us into familiar places, whose stories are well worn and well told. As we remember and embody those stories through our movements, we can ask: What comes up for us? What do we remember? What haven't we remembered until that moment?

Asana is not

- only physical exercise or a weight-loss program
- a competitive sport
- yoga unless it encompasses pranayama and meditation
- only for cisgendered, thin, white, wealthy women

Asana is

- an embodied spiritual practice
- a way to prepare the body for the rigors of meditation
- a practice to align the body, mind, and heart
- in service to uncovering and releasing the stories that live within us
- available to all bodies in all shapes, sizes, and abilities

⁘ Asana Reflection Questions

It's important to make time for asana or movement practices that connect you with your physical body every day. Part of practicing asana is learning to feel into and trust your soma, to experience what autonomy in movement feels like, and how to take your seat of power and presence. Here are a few questions to consider:

For the Self

- As you practice, notice the places in your body that feel tight or constricted, the places that feel particularly open, and the places you may have neglected. Now, allow the breath to take you into where you feel most grounded and powerful. Move from that sense of stability and ease. As you come out, consider writing in a journal or jotting down a few notes. What did you notice? Were you able to stay connected to the intention of groundedness as you moved?
- As you practice your asana, notice which stories emerge. Where do they live in your body? What did you need to do to create more space for them to surface?
- Choose your favorite pose. What effects does it have on the other four koshas or bodies (energy, mental, wisdom, and bliss)?
- How can you take small micro steps to make time for asana or movement practices each day?

With Others

- It's often said that when we do yoga, the world becomes a kinder, gentler place. What do you think that means? How does your asana practice affect the people around you?
- How does it feel to practice yoga in a studio setting with other students? How does that differ from doing asana at home?
- Practice observing the messages, stories, and communications that happen nonverbally when you practice asana with others. Where can you create and make space within you so you can be in a state of receptivity and openness to the body wisdom coming through others?

In the World

- How can your individual soma support the development and nourishment of soma in the world?
- How does doing asana help you connect to your community?
- How can you invite embodied movement into communities committed to equality and social justice?
- Where can you expand the physical possibilities for yourself and others to have bodily autonomy and freedom?

∷ ASANA PRACTICE

Here's a short yoga sequence that supports spiritual nourishment and connection to that which is greater than you and integration with yourself, your community, and the world. This sequence is slow and nourishing with options for support in earth-based practice. Together we will practice connection and grounding.

With options in each shape, it also creates awareness and extension in your body to help you maintain ahimsa through powerful choices in movement for self-care. It ends with a simple relaxation to integrate. The more nurturance you bring to yourself, the more you can take the practice of ahimsa out into your community and world.

Yoga is a spiritual practice from India that aims at liberation—it is here for all of us. Remember, yoga is not a competition; it's an experience. Each shape may look and feel different, from person to person, even from one side of the body to another. Let me be a guide and your body, mind, spirit be the authority. During this practice, allow yourself to feel active rest, surrender, and kindness in as many shapes and movements as possible.

The Sequence

Bring your mind, body, and heart together as you join your hands at the center of your chest in Anjali mudra. Take three deep breaths, in and out.

Listen inward for groundedness and truth and move with an open mind and heart.

Draw your attention inward and downward into all the parts of you touching the earth. Allow your breath to move easefully and slowly. If your breath gets stuck, slow down to let it glide as you move.

Inhale and raise your arms up any amount away from the earth.

Exhale and lower your arms any amount toward the earth.

Inhale and twist your torso to one side.

Exhale and twist deeper.

Inhale and return to center.

Inhale and twist your torso to the other side.

Exhale and twist deeper.

Inhale and return to center.

Exhale and fold forward any amount toward the earth.

Let your body move toward the earth feeling grounded support.

Inhale and rise.

Exhale and relax.

May I let my consciousness rest and restore itself through practices such as asana.

May my body, mind, and spirit be at peace.

SADHAKAS SPEAK: TEJAL PATEL

Each day is a bit different. More so now than ever before, which in large part is due to the shifting global and local landscape created by the ongoing pandemic. My sadhana has adjusted to this unraveling of routine and I'm comforted by seated meditation, slow flows, quiet moments with a warm cup of chai, and deep nourishing conversations with like-minded friends.

I've leaned into the world of online practice and have enjoyed engaging when it best suits me. I think it's a new day for moving away from regimented times for practice, as it feels like the less structure we have in most things provides an opportunity for space, deep rest, and openness for collaboration without resistance.

My sadhana has always been my safe harbor, moving my body has always brought me solace, and finding moments of quiet in my mind has always brought me closer to peace. I've continued to allow my practice to undulate as needs be, whether I'm flowing and breathing alone, with others; reading; journaling; creating and envisioning; or responding. In these waves of constant change I am grateful to be on this path.

—Tejal Patel, yoga teacher, community
organizer, podcaster

Pranayama: The Breath within the Breath

"There is no yoga without the breath" is a saying I've heard countless times. And it's true. Of course, there is no *life* without the breath either! Luckily the breath is controlled by the autonomic nervous system, which means we breathe whether we're conscious of it or not. Although we don't have to worry about remembering to breathe, we *can* actively take control of our breath whenever we want to. We can slow it down by focusing on the exhalation when we're anxious, or enliven it by expanding the inhalation when we feel lethargic. We do that through the practice of pranayama, the fourth limb of Raja Yoga. *Pranayama* combines *prana*, meaning "energy" or "life force," with either *yama*, "control" or "restraint," or *ayama*, "extension" or "expansion." Paradoxically, both are useful. Pranayama techniques put us in touch with our breath and give us an opportunity to consciously control it, which often means expanding it into the areas of our body that need attention.

Western science has studied the effects of pranayama on the

autonomic and central nervous systems and offers a physiological explanation of its power: slowing down the breath activates the parasympathetic nervous system and promotes a sense of relaxation, calm, and increased comfort and decreases anxiety, depression, and anger. While it's nice to have Western science validate what yogis have known for millennia, in reality, pranayama is more than just the breath moving in and out of our lungs. Pranayama is the breath within the breath; our vital life-force energy that brings oxygen and vitality to every cell in our body. It connects us to the *koshas*—the deeper and subtler aspects of ourselves, including our thinking mind and our wisdom or intuitive mind. Breathing exercises serve an essential purpose in Hatha Yoga practice; they help us pay close attention to our bodily functions and energy flow. Pranayama techniques can relax or energize; calm the mind or wake it up; cool the body down or warm it up; create mental serenity or intensity. Deep breathing allows us to stretch the body more consciously, which can help prevent injury. Breath practices also rejuvenate and stimulate bodily systems through the release of dormant energy. On a physical level, practicing pranayama can also contribute to lowering blood pressure, relieving anxiety, expanding capacity in your lungs, and sharpening the mind's focus.

Too often yoga in the West focuses solely on asana and leaves little to no time for pranayama or meditation. By doing this, asana becomes simply a fitness practice and its deeper and subtler benefits are elusive. Remember . . . no breath, no yoga!

Pranayama is not
- just an add-on to your asana practice—it is a vital aspect of yoga practice
- just mindful breathing
- forcefully controlling the breath

Pranayama is
- a way to notice what's happening in the body
- a way to heal the body and restore balance to the central nervous system and entire soma

- a way to increase our ability to connect with the subtle body and connect with life force

⠿ PRANAYAMA REFLECTION QUESTIONS

Adding pranayama and conscious breathing techniques to our daily practice brings our mind into places in the body that are asking for relief, love, and connection. Mind and breath work together.

For the Self
- Ask yourself: How is my breath right now? Is it long, short, smooth, choppy? Without changing it, simply bring awareness to breath.
- Notice how the rhythm of your breath changes in response to different feelings—sadness, anger, anxiety, joy. What did you discover? Write it down.
- What kinds of actions can you take to increase your capacity to breathe?

With Others
- Invite an intention for this moment. Can you breathe from a place of spaciousness and care for yourself and others?
- In placing your attention on the breath, how does it change the way you receive feedback or comments from people in your life?

In the World
- The way we breathe can impact the nervous systems of those around us. Try organizing a group breathe with friends or members of your community. How did the experience change the dynamic of the group? What were some reactions (including your own) to the practice?
- See if you can tune in to the collective breath in a room. Notice when folks are holding their breath. See if you can sync your breath with others. Take deep full breaths and slow your breathing down. What did it feel like to all breathe

together? How did it change the group dynamic or the energy in the room?

‼ PRANAYAMA PRACTICE

Here's a sweet pranayama to calm your mind and body and focus on balance, grounding, and strength building. The more deeply you breathe, the more care you bring to yourself—and the more you can take that care out into your community and world.

With pranayama, keep in mind this is not a competition but an experience. No body and no breath are the same. Your breath may feel different from inhale to exhale. In this exploration, let me be a guide and your body, mind, spirit be the main teacher. During this practice, allow yourself to feel active kindness in as many moments and breaths as possible.

Bring your mind, body, and heart together as you join your hands at the center of your chest in Anjali mudra. Take three deep breaths, in and out. Let your hands rest down in your lap and find an easeful way to be.

The Sequence

Draw your attention inward to where you notice your breathing.

Where do you notice it? At the tip of your nostrils? the inner part of your nose? the back of your throat? your upper chest? your abdomen or belly?

Can you feel your breath moving your body—perhaps lifting your shoulders, expanding your ribs, or softening your belly?

Bring your awareness to a single point of focus on your breath.

Notice your in-breath and your out-breath.

As you inhale, notice the length of your inhale.

As you exhale, notice the length of your exhale.

Become aware of the pause at the end of your inhale.

Become aware of the pause at the end of your exhale.

Without needing to change or control your breath, simply allow your awareness to rest upon it.

Continue to practice like this for as long as you are able: five, ten, fifteen, or thirty minutes.

If your mind wanders, bring it back with kindness, joy, and gratitude. When you notice it wandering, you can return to focus on your breath. Enjoy!   ⁑

PRATYAHARA: DRAWING THE SENSES INWARD

Pratyahara plays a transitional role within the eight limbs, moving us from the external to the internal and back again. In an article for *Yoga International* magazine, the author and Vedic teacher David Frawley points out that it's almost impossible for most of us to go directly from asana to meditation without getting control over—and developing—the breath and the senses. He goes on to say, "This is where pranayama and pratyahara come in. With pranayama we control our vital energies and impulses, and with pratyahara we gain mastery over the unruly senses—both prerequisites to successful meditation."[2] Through pratyahara we begin to absorb the fruits of our practice, not as specific exercises or steps but as part of who we are. It prepares us for the deeper work of liberation by teaching us to gather our senses and draw them increasingly inward to reduce external distractions so the mind can rest in a calm and receptive state.

The word pratyahara means against (*prati*) food (*ahara*). I'm happy to report that being "against food" doesn't imply that we have to stop eating to realize liberation. "Food" in this case means anything you take into your body, mind, or heart through your sense organs—your ears, eyes, nose, tongue, and skin. So pratyahara essentially means not being controlled by what you experience from the outside world.

Patanjali describes three levels of *ahara*. The first is obvious—the actual food you eat; how you care for and nourish your body. The second is sensory impressions—what you hear, smell, taste, touch, and see. The third is association—what you take in from others, mentally and emotionally. Pratyahara is the practice of turning your focus away from anything that does not nourish your mind, body, or heart and does not foster connection. At the same time, pratyahara helps quiet the mind enough so that you can turn *toward* what truly nourishes you.

Resting deeply while enjoying a clear mind requires us to detach ourselves from the external world. This does not mean that we completely lose contact with outer reality. This simply means we do not let ourselves be disturbed or distracted by our sensory experiences. It's like the feeling of having an itch but not needing to scratch it. Or hearing a sound but not needing to investigate it. Being aware without reacting. Pratyahara can be done in relaxation poses such as *savasana* (corpse pose), in an active asana practice, and even in daily life situations. My personal pratyahara practice makes me a kinder, more present, and more attuned person. By consciously withdrawing into a quieter state of being first, I am able to respond to the external world with more discernment and less attachment.

Pratyahara is *not* an invitation to stop seeing, hearing, or feeling what is happening all around you. It means getting quiet enough to pay attention, to withdraw *from* the world in order to *draw back in* without distortion (satya) and with compassion (ahimsa). You are still aware of the sounds, smells, tastes, and the sensation on your skin. But you don't try to identify where they come from; you don't reach out to grab them—you just allow them to move into your awareness and then you let them go. For example, you may hear birdsong as you practice. Instead of wondering where the sound is coming from, what type of bird it is, and what it's doing, you simply receive the sound without interruption or interpretation. In this way, pratyahara can also help intensify your connection to the yamas and niyamas, as well as your asana and pranayama practice. Asana, pranayama, and pratyahara do not happen singularly or in a vacuum. Taken together, they progressively move us deeper into our body, our breath, and our sensory gates. They give us information about ourselves, one another, and the world, helping us notice when we are out of sync and how that feels in the body.

Pratyahara is not

- an escape from the world
- shirking responsibilities
- focusing only on yourself

Pratyahara is

- a way of fine-tuning one's sensory focus
- practices to deepen awareness of self and world
- focusing inward to be more present within and all around

⣿ Pratyahara Reflection Questions

Periodically, throughout your day, stop and allow the sights, sounds, and smells around you to come into your mind without trying to identify them or figure out where they're coming from or what they mean. Consider these questions:

For the Self

- How might you use your pratyahara practice to reduce distractions so you can home in on how you want to focus in your personal life and your work?
- Try practicing pratyahara at the end of your asana practice, while in savasana. How does that change your experience?

With Others

- How can pratyahara help you prioritize what you focus on in your relationships?
- How can pratyahara help deepen your practice and commitment to the yamas?

In the World

- What kinds of actions can you take to create a world that sees and acknowledges your presence rather than focusing on what is absent or what you lack?
- What kind of actions can you take to create a world in which you see and acknowledge others?

:: Pratyahara Practice

Here's a pratyahara practice that can help you draw the senses inward so you can focus your mind without distraction—and not completely shut out the external world. The more you bring your attention gently inward, the more focused care you bring to yourself—and the more you can take that care out into your community and world.

With pratyahara, remember it's a matter of *abhyasa* (practice) and *vairagya* (nonattachment) as well, so don't be too hard on yourself. When you lose focus, just gently come back and begin again, knowing that each time you do, you are planting seeds of concentration that will lead to insight. In this exploration, let me be a guide and your own body, mind, and spirit be the main teacher. During this practice, allow yourself to feel active kindness in as many moments of focus as possible.

Bring your mind, body, and heart together as you join your hands at the center of your chest in Anjali mudra. Take three deep breaths, in and out.

Listen with an open mind and heart.

May I draw my attention inward, reducing *vrittis*, which are fluctuations of thought or disturbances in the mind.
May I explore meditative states of consciousness that support my peace.
May I be mindful of the food that I eat and be nourishing for my mind, body, and spirit.
May I let my consciousness rest and restore itself through practices such as yoga nidra or restorative yoga.
May my sense impressions be at peace.   ::

SADHAKAS SPEAK: DIVYA BALAKRISHNAN

∷

My journey with yoga has been multifold. Over decades it guided me through growing pains, heartache, social justice, and personal liberation. My yoga sadhana began with consistency and intensity as the cornerstones of my practice. It seemed like the more rigorous my practice of asana was, the sooner I would become a master at yoga as a whole. Opening myself up to the full expression of yoga was the key to understanding where my study needed to grow.

Today my practice centers around a deep-rooted ritual of self-compassion. I always begin with an honest look at my current state—emotional, physical, and mental. This becomes the foundation upon which I use the limbs of yoga like building blocks. On any given day I may need a few moments of meditation upon waking to set an intention for the rest of the day—a grounding point to return to whenever I begin to feel removed from myself.

There are multiple points of study throughout the week, wherein I read about mudras or practice pranayama or study philosophical texts. There is always movement—careful, intentional, and compassionate. Over time, this manner of practicing yoga becomes my sadhana.

—Divya Balakrishnan, E-RYT 200 educator
and teacher trainer

5

Dharana, Dhyana, and Samadhi

Mapping the Inner Landscape

WE NOW MOVE into the last triad of Patanjali's yogic Eightfold Path—dharana (concentration), dhyana (meditation), and samadhi (absorption). These three inner limbs, when practiced together, are called *sanyam* (to control or integrate), and they move us deeper into the meditative state of absorption. As the yoga teacher and healer Nischala Joy Devi points out in her unique commentary on the Yoga Sutras, these three aren't *practices* per se; rather, they are "states that blossom through the nurturing practices that precede them."[1] I agree. I can't imagine trying to corral my mind into any kind of meditative state without my asana, pranayama, and pratyahara practices.

As explained in the previous chapter, we approach our internal landscape after we've refined bahiranga, the external one. We've used asana to help prepare our body for deeper practices by strengthening and grounding our physical container. We've practiced pranayama to release any stuckness that prevents our vital life force from expanding into all parts of the body. And our pratyahara practice has moved the mind further inward, disentangling the senses from the experiences they actively seek outside of the body.

DHARANA: COLLECTING THE MIND

Once the mind lets go of what no longer serves it and the senses settle into contentment, we can begin to gather, or "yoke," the senses so that we can fix our full attention on one thing. This is dharana, the practice of concentration—the first step toward experiencing meditation (dhyana) and, ultimately, unconditional love and abiding peace (samadhi).

The mind isn't always an easy thing to "collect," which can make any meditative or concentration practice a challenge—and for most of us, even a *lifelong* challenge. In the Yoga Sutras, Patanjali mentions five different states of mind or consciousness, called *citta bhumis*. The first one, *kshipta bhumi*, is the distracted mind, the monkey mind, which flits from thing to thing and is impossible to corral. *Mudha bhumi* is the dull, sleepy, what's-the-point mind, which is often accompanied by depression and sadness. *Vikshipta bhumi* is the partially focused mind, which has moments of clarity and concentration but gets pulled away easily. Some liken it to a butterfly that alights on a flower, stays for the sweetness, and off it goes again to the next pretty thing. *Ekagra bhumi* is the single-pointed mind, which is fully focused on the object it has chosen. The fifth bhumi, *niruddha*, is the state in which the fluctuations of the mind have been stilled and the mind is in a state of pure awareness.[2] All five states of mind benefit from contemplative practices, including yoga nidra, pratyahara, dharana, and dhyana.

Ekagra bhumi is the state of mind that is developed through dharana. Practicing dharana means to concentrate fully on a single point—either with your eyes, ears, or voice—and keep it there, allowing everything else to fall away. That single point can be anything. You can choose an external object for your focus, such as a candle flame, flower, statue of a god or goddess, or photo of a spiritual teacher. You can choose an internal object, such as the point between your eyebrows, the palms of your hands, the lotus within your heart (where your personal ishvara resides), or your breath. Or you can rest your full attention on a mantra or a phrase that you repeat silently or chant aloud. Regardless of what you choose, by holding your mind within a center of spiritual consciousness, dharana allows you to stay in present-moment awareness, connected to the truth within.

Your focus point is called your *drishti*. The ancients believed (and rightly so) that where our gaze is directed, our attention naturally follows; and that the quality of our gaze is directly reflected in the quality of our thoughts. Like a mantra, a drishti is a cradle that supports the mind. When the gaze is fixed on a single point *within* the body, your attention draws inward and the mind remains undisturbed by external stimuli. The use of a drishti allows the mind to hold its focus, moving from vikshipta bhumi, partially focused or "butterfly" mind, to ekagra bhumi and into a deeper state of concentration.

It's important not to strain the eyes or the brain during dharana practice. Keep your eyes soft and your facial muscles relaxed. Of course, for most of us, it can be pretty impossible to place our undivided attention on a single object for an extended period of time. By extended, I mean more than three or four breaths or maybe even a minute on a "good" day! Dharana is definitely a challenge—but it is not meant to be a *mental* challenge. You're not trying to fix or figure anything out. There's nothing to solve. To be in a state of dharana is to *rest* in concentrated awareness, *not* to strain or struggle; to patiently invite your attention to move back to the breath and then back to its focus. Patanjali calls this abhyasa, a gentle reminder to return over and over and over again to your practice, coupled with vairagya, an invitation to loosen the grip on what that practice must look like and even what you're *supposed to* gain.

Dharana is not
- forcing your mind to focus
- a meditation practice per se; it is a practice to train the mind
- different brain-training exercises for better stamina
- a practice intended to make us better producers and consumers in capitalist society

Dharana is
- discovering the essential nature of an object
- a concentration practice to focus the mind
- complete absorption into an object
- losing a sense of time, space, place, and separation
- entering a flow state

‫❖‬ Dharana Reflection Questions

Dharana opens our perceptions beyond what we had ever imagined possible. Dharana is also quite a practical, present-moment practice! Who doesn't want to be more focused, less scattered? To be able to home in on a task or a conversation with laser-like attention? In considering the role that dharana practice can play in your life, here are some questions:

For the Self

- How does choosing a particular drishti during your asana practice change your experience?
- Try practicing dharana by choosing different points of focus—mantra, mudra, breath, and visualization. How did each one feel? Did you feel drawn to one in particular?
- How can practicing concentration help your meditation practice?

With Others

- Think back on a time when you found yourself completely "in the moment," absorbed in an action or a conversation that caused you to lose contact with time and place. What were you doing? What did that feel like? What kinds of activities move you into the "flow"?
- Using the single-pointed attention of dharana, how does that change your day-to-day experiences? What would it look like to bring dharana into a relationship—with your partner, your child, or in a friendship?

In the World

- How comfortable are you with practicing dharana in any and every moment? With mindfulness, can everything be a possible place of practice?
- How can practicing dharana in a group setting support your practice and help you stay the course?

❖ Two Dharana Practices

Mantra

Choose a mantra for today's practice. It could be the sound of your breath, perhaps, the *shhh* of the inhale and exhale; SO HUM; SHANTI, SHANTI, PEACE, PEACE; or any phrase that gives you a sense of calm. Once you choose, let your mind and body rest into the mantra. Begin to embody your mantra by coordinating your breath with its sound or phrase (example: inhale SO, exhale HUM. Or inhale "in," exhale "out"). If you find your mind wandering—and you will!—kindly and gently notice it and return to the mantra along with your breath. By holding the mind on a mantra and practicing deeply, dharana allows us to stay in present-moment awareness, connected to the truth within us.

Practice like this quietly for three to five minutes, gently bringing the mind back to the present whenever it wanders off. Notice the effects on your senses and gently ease back into your day.

Drishti

Light a candle and gaze at it for two to three minutes. No matter how focused your mind is on that candle flame, thoughts or feelings may bubble up to the surface. Simply notice them, smile, and let them go. Some days you may be able to calm your thoughts and focus your mind a little easier; other days, not so much. Feel free to focus on the third eye, the point within your body between and slightly above the eyebrows.

> This tapas, heat, or concentration of mind creates the
> yoga practice.
> —YOGA SUTRA[3]   ❖

DHYANA: MEDITATIVE AWARENESS

Maintaining a focus that is clear and vast, resting your awareness in the integrated universal spirit, is known as meditation, or dhyana, the second of the three inner limbs. It is where time exists—even a

single moment—without the ego's preferences or resistance. No longer are we running away, reaching to grasp, spacing out, or bracing
for impact. In fact, all fluctuations of the mind cease. This is the state
of uninterrupted bliss, and it can be achieved through the progressive practices of asana, pranayama, pratyahara, and dharana.

Dhyana is the second level of deep inner awareness, which can
lead to complete liberation (moksha) or enlightenment (samadhi).
While dharana is a meditative effort that trains the mind to focus
solely and steadily on a single object, dhyana is *effortless* meditation
in which the mind naturally moves toward the object—without having to focus on it, analyze it, judge it, name it, or attach meaning to
it—and becomes completely absorbed in it.

Practicing dhyana brings a heightened sense of awareness to your
practice that can result in moments of mental clarity, stillness, and
silence. When you become engrossed in whatever you're doing,
fully and without effort or force, you are firmly planted in the here
and now and there is no difference between the doing and the doer.
This type of present-moment mindfulness is a state of *being* achieved
when the attention naturally rests on the breath, a particular sound,
a sensation in the body, or a special place in nature. Dhyana builds
on dharana because dharana is an entryway into experiences of
deep meditation. You may experience this entry when you walk, eat,
or sit; when you move through an asana sequence or chant a mantra. It can look like a body scan, yoga nidra, deep relaxation, walking
in nature, or sitting in silence with eyes soft or lids closed.

Dhyana supports us when we feel uneasy, confused, or reactive
by teaching us to pause, allow our attention to move into the body,
and collect ourselves before speaking or acting. This can be especially helpful before addressing conflict in our personal, social, and
professional worlds.

Dhyana is not
- a technique to empty or control your mind
- a concentration practice
- daydreaming or a way to let your mind wander
- complete enlightenment and detachment from this world

Dhyana is
- moving into stillness
- a clear, untroubled mind
- realization in this world in this moment
- a state of being in which there is no separation between you and what you're focusing on

⁘ DHYANA REFLECTION QUESTIONS

Dhyana gives us a taste of what it means to become fully immersed in the present moment, to experience a sense of unity with all beings. It brings clarity to the mind and compassion into the heart. Consider these questions as you practice:

For the Self
- Have you ever experienced a deep meditative state of aware-ness—even for a moment? Where were you—at home, in nature, in the presence of another? What were the conditions that brought you there?
- Is there a particular place or type of practice you find brings you more peace? Can you go there in your mind and notice how it changes how you're feeling right now?

With Others
- Have you ever meditated with people you're close to? What was that like? Was it different from meditating on your own? If so, how?
- How does a daily meditation practice enhance the relation-ships you have with your family, partner, and community?

In the World
- How can consistent meditation practice help you become aware of emotions—or put out the fire—within yourself so you can be present, listen, and even attend to the needs of others?

- How can dhyana practice lead to compassion for the suffering of others—for example, those who experience systemic and cultural inequities?
- How can trauma-informed and consent-based meditation practices within community organizations help enhance their work in the world?

⁞⁞ DHYANA PRACTICE: MOVING INTO STILLNESS

Create a solid foundation by feeling your sitz bones on the surface where you are. Align your spine. Send your head up toward the sky.

Allow your attention to rest on the breath. As you breathe in, notice your breath moving in. As you breathe out, notice the breath moving out. In, out. In, out.

Notice your thoughts like clouds as they float by. Your mind is like the clear blue sky behind the clouds. No matter what thoughts or clouds float by, your consciousness is vast and open like the clear, blue sky.

It is natural for the mind to wander. The point is not to completely empty the mind but to bring your mind back gently and kindly to your breath. Feel the openness and expansiveness of your mind's open awareness.

Practice this several times a week, if possible, until you can sit for three to five minutes and are able to feel a sense of calm abiding. ⁞⁞

SADHAKAS SPEAK: JESAL PARIKH

⁞⁞

I practice yoga every day. But my sadhana doesn't look how you'd expect it to look. For the last few years, my practice has become less structured and more fluid. In the morning I awaken to the sound of the Gayatri Mantra, a sacred Vedic chant practiced for thousands of years to invoke enlightenment, wisdom, and awakening (something I've been doing for over a decade), and I just listen and take in the vibration as I start my day. I practice pranayama and *mantra japa*, the meditative practice of repeating a mantra, often while using a mala or prayer beads to focus the mind and as a way to tap into my inner power. To my surprise, mantra japa has become a frequent practice that helps me through many challenging situations. I sometimes practice asanas. I try to exercise daily, and whether I'm weightlifting, boxing, or cycling, I always incorporate mindfulness as part of the practice. But either way, I never skip savasana or my ahimsa and aparigraha work—kindness to myself and nonattachment to the outcome of the practice or workout I've just done. And trust me, for someone like me who isn't naturally athletic, it's not an easy thing to disrupt self-criticism and practice gratitude for my body in the moment. Meditation most often comes in the form of daily walks with my dog, when I leave my phone at home and remind myself over and over to stay present to my surroundings. I also often practice a few minutes of *vipassana* meditation, a focus of observing my thoughts, emotions, and bodily sensations, before bed or do body relaxation exercises to help me fall asleep. My most cherished practice, however, is svadhyaya—the study of yogic philosophy and how it applies to me in a way that makes me get out of my own way so that life flows that much smoother.

—Jesal Parikh, yoga industry disrupter

Samadhi: Present-Moment Bliss

The seven limbs of Raja Yoga that we've been exploring have led us to the experience of samadhi. Samadhi is described as a state of complete union in which the individual merges with the divine or universal consciousness. There is no longer a "me and mine." No separate ego. No "other." There is only a sense of fullness within emptiness. This integration, or union, is believed to be the true expression of the eternal self, without form or end. What is it, then, that we are united with or absorbed into? Some call this union the Self, Life, God, the Force, Brahma, or simply "All That Is." Use whatever words resonate with your heart; to fully describe the experience of complete union is beyond language or verse.

In the Yoga Sutras, Patanjali gets very specific about the many different stages of samadhi and what we need to do to achieve each one. Remember, though, Patanjali's audience were renunciates on the path to transcend life, to realize moksha—complete liberation from the cycle of birth, death, and rebirth. Chances are it's not our immediate goal, as householders, to transcend the physical plane. Nonetheless, samadhi is achievable in this lifetime. My teacher, Shankarji, says samadhi is *not* something far away or something we can only attain when we pass from this life. Samadhi is a state of being that can happen in a single moment—and it can melt away just as quickly!

So what *does* it mean to experience samadhi in the twenty-first century? Let's start by defining the word. *Sama* means "equal" or "even," and *dhi* means "intellect." *Samadhi* can be translated as "equanimity," "standing in the middle," or "seeing equally." When you're in a state of equanimity, you transcend the intellect—that which differentiates—and you see only union, connection, oneness. You experience life *as it is* without judgment, without discriminating. It is that moment when you realize there is no separation between you and any other being. When you begin to understand that you are both the oppressor and the oppressed—the cause of suffering *and* the one who suffers—you have entered into a state of *being* instead of a state of *doing*.

You may get a taste of samadhi during pranayama, whenever you drop into an extended pause between your exhale and inhale. In that pause there are no thoughts and no thinker, no reactions and no person reacting—only silence and stillness; a feeling of complete absorption in the moment. Samadhi can also happen in nature when you overwhelmingly feel connected to everything around you. You may also experience samadhi when you encounter a stranger or connect with a friend and realize you share the same emotions— even without necessarily sharing the same experience—and that you both have the same needs: to be loved and to not suffer.

Samadhi as the Power of Insight in the Present Moment

Powerful insights naturally arise when you move through the eight limbs of Raja Yoga, particularly the three inner limbs. When the mind settles into stillness, your yoga practice can bring great insights and moments of true clarity, which allow you to cut through all kinds of suffering, including fear, despair, anger, and discrimination.

Insight comes from deep understanding. If we don't take time to be mindful, focus our drishti, and concentrate, insight will not manifest in us. It's important to create the kind of environment where mindfulness and concentration become easy. It's like preparing the soil so that the flower you plant can sprout. Insight is an intuitive inner knowing that comes from practicing yoga and honing your mindfulness. This inner knowing, or insight, is built upon the foundation of regular practice and focused awareness. If you allow yourself to get lost in regrets about the past or worries about the future, it will be difficult to grow insight and to know what right action to take in the present. Poetically, samadhi is that moment when fire and ice, movement and stillness, the rose, thorn, and wholeness of the entire plant become one.

I had my own samadhi moment after a daily practice session. I was sitting in meditation and as my breath slowed down to a steady rhythm, I suddenly became aware of the earth spinning around the sun, the movement of the sun itself, the solar system and all of the energies and essences in it. I experienced a feeling of absolute convergence—all things coming together. In that moment I felt the smallness of my human experience in the context of the great ebbing and flowing of energy through time and space. But I didn't feel sad or alone or pointless. I felt completely connected to everything around me and beyond me. I knew enough about sadhana not to try to hold on to the experience. I allowed it to arise, be with me and I with it, and dissolve. We became one. I can't say how long I was there. It could have been a single moment or several, an hour or even more. Eventually the feeling faded. But it left within me a residue of that feeling of interconnectedness. After that experience I didn't feel so alone in the world anymore because I had had a visceral, embodied experience of interconnectedness, an awareness of the pure joy and bliss available to me. In many practice sessions and even throughout everyday life, I get touches and tastes of this experience.

Samadhi isn't something to strive for outside of ourselves. In fact, it's not really a "thing." It's a state of being that is available to all of us here and now. When we experience it, it imbues our everyday life with joy, purpose, and meaning.

Samadhi is not
- a technique you can *practice* and get better at
- something you achieve once and forever
- something that separates you from the world
- the same as self-realization

Samadhi is
- an embodied experience of self and world as completely interconnected; a sense of presence in which you feel connected and not alone
- often experienced through metaphor or symbol, such as waves, energies, movement, or profound stillness
- the interconnection of one's small-s self with the big-S Self!
- complete oneness; the realization that there is no separation between you and another
- *citta vritti nirodhah*—the resting of the mind into stillness—the ultimate goal of spiritual practice immersed in equanimity

❖❖ SAMADHI REFLECTION QUESTIONS

Holding the great bow of yogic wisdom, the aspirant should fix the arrow of mind, sharpened with meditation, on its target. Draw the string with full absorption and shoot at the target. My friend, remember immutable, eternal Truth alone is the target.

—*Mundaka Upanishad*

For the Self
- What are three small ways that you can deepen self-acceptance and joy?
- Have you ever experienced a time during meditation—sitting, walking, or chanting—when you became fully absorbed in the silence? When there was no separation between you and your surroundings? What did that feel like?
- What insights have emerged through a committed practice of *samyama* (the simultaneous practice and experience of dharana, dhyana, and samadhi)?

With Others
- How can your awareness of interbeing and interdependence support you in the practice of uplifting one another's liberation?
- Describe a time when you felt completely absorbed in the moment with another person. What did that feel like? What were you doing? What did you notice?

In the World
- What would it feel like to live as if anything other than union were just an illusion? How would that change how you show up in the world?
- In practicing samyama, how has that enhanced, changed, or otherwise influenced your commitment to alleviating suffering?

⠃⠃ SAMADHI PRACTICE

Samadhi is not something you can practice to "get good at." It's a state of being you sometimes just fall into. One of the best ways to prepare the mind and the body to experience this state of undifferentiated bliss is to faithfully practice the other seven limbs of yoga, incorporating them into your life. And then pay attention. Another important outcome of the trifecta practice of dharana, dhyana, and samadhi is a commitment to selfless service, the understanding that no one is free until we are all free; that we must do all we can to alleviate the suffering of others. From meditation or practice on our mat to welcoming people into our studios and classrooms, we can practice yoga as transformation of trauma—yoga as healing and unity.

This can be our yoga-unity check-in as we bring this practice of yoga into our personal, family, community, and social world, appreciating those moments of unity and oneness as they occur and grow.   ⠃⠃

In part 2 we explore what it means to walk a spiritual path with yoga as our guide; to choose life as a sadhaka and commit wholeheartedly to social justice and selfless service. May this path challenge you. May it inspire you. May it lead you back to your own inner wisdom.

Part Two
Heeding the Sadhaka's Call

Even if you have known the real truth you have to practice always.

—Yoga Vashistha

6

Becoming an Agent
of Spiritual Possibility
Yoga as Spiritual Practice

The wise one beholds all beings in the Self and the Self in
all beings; for that reason he uplifts all.

—*ISHA UPANISHAD*

YOGA ISN'T YOGA until it's personal, until you take the teachings
into your heart and make them your own. Yoga becomes a spiritual practice when you allow it to move through you, when you can
breathe into it, feel, hear, taste, and touch its presence. Yoga helps
us to know ourselves intimately, a crucial first step in knowing how
to be in relationship with others. This journey inward begins in the
body and invites us to peel back the layers to discover the secrets
that lie within. The challenge for many practitioners in the West
is that their yoga practice stops with the physical body. Instead of
being just one aspect of yoga, asana has been misrepresented as synonymous with fitness and outward appearances in the West for close
to eighty years, giving it a position of outsized importance. Many of
us have worked hard to put asana in its place within the larger context of spiritual inquiry. As a result, more and more teacher-training
programs, workshops, and retreats include the other seven limbs, as
well as spiritual texts and deeper practices. All of this is good!

Yet over the years I've noticed something interesting. Too often
folks intent on developing a spiritual practice don't see asana as
part of that. It becomes something separate—something they *do* to

strengthen their body, gain flexibility, relieve their sciatica, or cure their anxiety. But here's what I know: asana is and should be an *integral* part of the sadhaka's journey. It is a spiritual practice itself; an act of devotion to the divine essence within us. A full-body mudra practice. A way of caring for and honoring our physical container. There is no specific sequence to memorize, equipment to purchase, or number of hours to devote. But there *is* something magical and powerful that happens when we realize that practice on our mat can feed and sustain our practice off the mat too. Committing to yoga as a spiritual practice, as your personal sadhana, begins by making yoga your own, by preserving the tenets of this ancient practice in a way that speaks to you.

For many in my family, we learned yoga as a way of life long before we learned to move our bodies into a sequence of shapes and postures. It's the way we *live*, something interwoven into the fabric of daily existence. It's what and how we eat, where we shop, how we handle conflict, and who we seek out for support. It's how we find calm and ease, how we worship, and how we express and feel inspiration. My *aita* (grandmother) Lakshmi Devi Barkataki embodied yoga in so many ways. She was, in turns, funny, serious, and strongly superstitious. She married and became a mother at age thirteen. Though she had many challenges and few material possessions, she was incredibly generous. She embodied *seva*, the yogic principle of selfless service. My father tells of growing up in their mud-walled home in Dibrugarh, Assam, and how everyone in the neighborhood knew his mother. She and her husband, Krishna Chandra Barkataki, were always quick to share what they had with anyone, regardless of caste or class, inviting those less fortunate to stay in their home and receive care and sustenance. Their practice of yoga was not something that they did only for an hour a day. It was their sadhana. Although they practiced puja and worshipped at certain times, yoga infused every moment of the waking day. It is who they are and what they do in the world.

Yoga is a living practice accessible to all of us. It yokes the ancient teachings to our modern lives, allowing us to lean back on authentic yoga culture as a vessel for shaping change in the present. It invites us to lean into its roots as we practice forward, choosing an authentic, embodied yoga that centers equity and spiritual fulfillment.

When you are confronted with challenges or you don't know which direction to go, yoga shines a light as you fumble around in the dark. Every few feet you move, you see a little clearer. Keep going, committed to your own unfolding. And always remember that the vehicle of yogic consciousness moves in us and through us to be shared with all beings.

As I've practiced, listened, and learned, I've felt that yoga is its own conscious being. It doesn't care what color you are, what culture you're from, what religion you affiliate with. It doesn't matter if you practice at a high-end resort, in a small apartment, or a tent high up in the Himalayas. Yoga just wants you to be in integrity and use it as it is intended: to yoke, to build bridges, and to dissolve separations within and without.

You've perhaps heard tales of a hero or heroine's journey, which is most often an epic external adventure. The mythologist and storyteller Joseph Campbell explores this framework in his work on the hero's journey in *The Hero with a Thousand Faces*.[1] The sadhaka embarks on an *internal* journey of personal transformation no less epic—an interplay between the self and other; a journey of interconnected transformation. Sadhakas are no longer dependent on the outside world for power or courage. They have awakened Shakti, the power that comes from within. Dwelling in a state of complete liberation, independence, and joy, they strive to make the world a better place for all beings. The journey begins internally and becomes external, and then there's no distinction between the two as we embody the unity and interconnection that yoga offers.

So what does it mean to commit to yoga as your personal sadhana, as something you can bring into your daily life? I believe it means to approach every moment as sacred; to set our *sankalpa*—a heartfelt, personal vow—"to manifest our deepest resolve to focus and act according to our physical, mental, emotional, and pranic capacity."[2] In other words, to become an agent of spiritual possibility.

BECOMING AN AGENT OF SPIRITUAL POSSIBILITY

When we bring yoga into our lives, we commit to a way of being in relationship with ourselves and others that is centered in love (ahimsa), truth (satya), and devotion (ishvara pranidhana). Three of the most important precepts in the yoga tradition, they inform how we think, speak, and act. Showing up in love and committing to deep listening and truthful engagement becomes a complete practice of devotion, a way of honoring the true teachings of yoga so that we can become agents of spiritual possibility—that is, spiritual changemakers.

The term *agents of spiritual possibility* is used by many change-making folks on the front lines who are actively working to disrupt cynicism, apathy, and inaction. They have found that their relentless hard work, frustration, anger, and grief are not enough to fuel effective and sustainable movements for change. They also realize that many of the challenges of our times cannot be solved with logic alone. We need heartfelt solutions for an interwoven humanity. We need ways of thinking about and solving problems that truly center the interconnectedness of all beings and are based in the understanding that there's no other way to see—or be in—the world. Agents of spiritual possibility apply spiritual technologies to fuel and sustain their hope, faith, belief, and work. Their optimism is *not* spiritual bypassing. They clearly see *and feel* the suffering and dire needs all around them and apply the teachings they have learned and embodied to make a difference.

As changemakers, we are encouraged to cultivate four positive mind states that can help us show up in love and minimize harm: loving-kindness, compassion, sympathetic joy, and equanimity. These mind states are found in all post-Vedic, Shramanic traditions, including in the Yoga Sutras, the Upanishads, Jain literature, and the Buddhist canon. Buddhists call them the four "immeasurables" (*brahmaviharas*) because they "represent love and goodwill toward all sentient beings, without limit."[3] In the Yoga Sutras (1:33) Patanjali writes,

Maitri karuna mudita upekshanam sukha duhka punya
apunya vishayanam bhavanatah chitta prasadanam.

Maitri (or *metta* in Pali) means "friendliness" or "loving-kindness."
Karuna is compassion. *Mudita* means "joyful uplift" or "sympathetic
joy." *Uppekha* means "equanimity," "standing in the middle," or nonattachment to results. Patanjali describes how in relationships, the
mind is brought to peace by embracing these practices. Universal
love is cultivated by feelings of friendliness toward those who are
happy, compassion for those who are suffering, goodwill toward
those who are virtuous, and neutrality toward those we experience
as unkind or adversarial.

What would it look like to put the *brahmaviharas* into practice as
an agent of spiritual possibility? How would that help you show up
in ways that are effective? Offering metta means that we love and
serve unconditionally, that our goodwill and benevolence go out
to all beings regardless of how we feel about them or whether we
agree with them. Karuna means that we feel the suffering of others
and vow to act in ways that can end or at least lessen it. Mudita is
delighting in the good fortune of others, even if it isn't *our* definition of good fortune. *Upeksha* is our commitment to "observe without interference" and not be searching for external validation when
we serve. We serve no matter what with an open heart and a listening ear.

Offering loving-kindness, compassion, and empathetic joy isn't
enough to effect change. Agents for spiritual possibility must also
work to uplift the underlying *causes* of happiness, find ways to alleviate the *causes* of suffering, participate in reducing harm and elevating
the comfort and happiness of others. In a wonderful article in *Tricycle* magazine, Theravadan Buddhist Thanissaro Bhikkhu describes
uppekha as a means of developing discernment, an important tool
for those of us involved in social justice.

Regardless of how strong your goodwill or compassion
may be, there are bound to be people whose past actions

are unskillful and who cannot or will not change their ways in the present. This is why you need equanimity as your reality check. When you encounter areas where you can't be of help, you learn not to get upset. Think about the universality of the principle of karma: it applies to everyone regardless of whether you like them or not. That puts you in a position where you can see more clearly what can be changed, where you can be of help. In other words, equanimity isn't a blanket acceptance of things as they are. It's a tool for helping you to develop discernment as to which kinds of suffering you have to accept and which ones you don't.[4]

GUIDELINES FOR LEADING THE SADHAKA WAY

••

- The essence of true service is to do no harm and to serve with love.
- Always show up in love and be open to learning.
- Listen for the truth, pay attention to what's underneath the words, and be open to multiple truths.
- Reflect back what you hear—and what the implications and intentions are—with curiosity and questions.
- Focus on process, not attainments.
- Dedicate the merits of your practice to something much bigger than yourself.

You can use yoga in your work as a changemaker without ever calling yourself (or becoming) a yoga teacher or leader. Being an agent of spiritual possibility, a caregiver in your world, a loving family member, an organizer and activist, a solid rock in your community—these are all ways to be of service with yoga. There are many examples of everyday changemakers who have relied on the foundations of yoga as they transform their lives and world. As we focus on a story or two, I invite you to think of your own story as well. I've seen teachers who work in the school system or in social services and use yoga to keep their calm and cool so that they can more readily serve hundreds of young people a day with kindness, compassion, and equanimity. Other teachers introduce the kids to mindfulness, yoga, and "brain breaks" during the school day. Still others help nonprofits understand the power of bringing ethics, discernment, and self-care into the work because they have seen how urgency can be used as a tool of white supremacy to disrupt the goals they're working toward. During times of political need, war and violence, yoga practitioners and teachers convene healing circles where community members can learn, grieve, listen, focus, and act.

We can also draw inspiration from the changemaking legacies past and present in yoga, such as the nonviolent social change movement that helped free India from British oppression. The movement was founded upon the yogic principles of ahimsa (nonviolence and love), satya (truth), and ishvara pranidhana (devotion to the divine) to form Satyagraha, or truth force. Through studying Gandhi's life, we know much of the emergence of this method founded on yogic philosophy, and there are many other people involved—whose names we may never know—who embodied the yogic principles of self- and community empowerment. Many of these freedom fighters took their inspiration from texts such as the Bhagavad Gita, as they fought for social change and developed a method that would later influence the Civil Rights Movement in the United States, the anti-apartheid movement in South Africa, the movement for decolonization, and scores of other movements for liberation and freedom around the world. Today, many movement leaders and participants continue to rely on yogic principles to drive their change work forward.

Some contemporary agents of spiritual possibility have become household names, including Arundhati Roy, the Booker Prize–winning writer who tells stories that would otherwise go untold as part of her lifelong activism; and the political activist and philosopher Angela Davis in her work in equity for Black liberation and feminism and the many decades she's spent speaking and teaching. There are thousands who are less well known sadhakas but no less important. Whether people know you and your efforts has no bearing on the spiritual foundation or the material impact of your work. You do not have to go out and do huge projects or be seen and recognized for what you do. You can be working on a small scale—local, person to person. Our work becomes spiritual when we honor and deeply value someone's agency and experience, when we show up in every aspect of our being; when we bring mindfulness and curiosity into all that we do and in doing so, create more harmony in the world. We each are part of the building blocks that make spiritual possibility and social change.

One example of a community working together as agents of spiritual possibility is a community group I was a part of in the early 2000s. I had just begun my work as a teacher at an under-resourced Title I public school in Los Angeles. Many of those who were graduating and working in support roles were queer young people who faced police and state violence as well as discrimination because of their gender identity, race, and class. We formed a kind of temporary family together. We built a community around shared needs. Who needs a place to live because their parents kicked them out for being queer? Whose sibling needed fundraising for bail funds or lawyer fees because they'd been incarcerated when they needed mental health treatment instead? We would get together and organize support for these needs.

We would always begin with a practice we called "Spiritual Space." This practice laid what we called a "spiritual foundation" for the service and equity work to come. We were a diverse group in terms of culture, race, age, and gender. So Spiritual Space might be an Ebo ceremony one day, a pagan ritual another day, or a Vedic meditation. Then we would strategize, organize, and plan. We would often cook and eat food together. Through these simple practices, always beginning with spiritual space as a foundation, we formed a community of spiritual social justice carers bringing art, meditation, organizing, beauty, and love into the world. We made revolution irresistible together. The spiritual space that we held together helped us understand one another, learn, and grow from the various wisdom traditions we each carried and that supported our work in the world. We celebrated many wins as a community—from bailing out family members and putting on art and fashion shows to raise funds for legal fees, to overturning policies that were harming our communities, such as truancy tickets for youth. We grieved many losses together as well, such as family members remaining behind bars or dying. Our spiritual practices supported us in working together to continue to create change.

We can't solve the problems of the world—or even within our intimate relationships—from breakdown. We must explore and work to solve our own and the world's problems from wholeness and connection. Which is to say, as agents of spiritual possibility, we must do the work of harmonizing our own nervous systems so that our brains can work in a whole, unified, optimal state. How do we do that? By centering self-care. For many of us, self-care has become synonymous with a capitalist fixation on buying our way to feeling good. The challenge with this reductionist belief is that self-care is seen as a form of self-indulgence, which only gets in the way of doing more and pushing harder. This is a sure recipe for burnout. The truth is, self-care is vital to our work, and yoga can support us in prioritizing it. Without self-care we run the risk of burning out. And nobody wants that. In chapter 15, we'll take a deeper look at what those self-care practices are and how they can move us from the brink of burnout to the balance we need to commit to social justice.

Are You a Spiritual Changemaker?

::

Your spiritual practice supports your compassion and
empathy in the work you do.
You work to align your actions with the principles of non-
harm, truth, and dedication.

You work to make yourself, your community, and the world better.

You center care for yourself as part of the work you do in the world.

You draw support from contemplative and spiritual practices as well as other changemakers.

You are open to collaboration with other spiritual changemakers.

You love to hear stories from—and applaud—other spiritual changemakers.

COMPASSION AND KINDNESS ARE KEY

As agents of spiritual possibility, we are committed to taking what we learn and using it for the benefit of others. We work to change hearts and minds from a spiritual foundation. As part of that foundation, we practice the yamas and niyamas, move our bodies and breathe in ways that ground and center our energy; we meditate, rest, and embrace joyful connection with others. All of this helps us recognize, experience, and be fully present to "what is" before we judge or even decide to add our voices to the conversation. Being fully present like this is a prerequisite to effective action, to conscious leadership in all forms. It requires a deep understanding and commitment to three yogic principles in particular: ahimsa, which invites us to do no harm and always lead with kindness, which is the cornerstone of ethical and conscious engagement; satya, which asks us to listen for, receive, and speak the truth; and ishvara pranidhana, which insists we put aside our egos and remember that we are not serving from a need to be right, acknowledged, or praised—we are serving with true devotion and selfless love. Practice noticing, acknowledging, and simply accepting the joy, humor, suffering, pain, sadness, and anger you see in yourself and others. Notice your breath, a powerful guide into presence: "Inhaling, I am present. Exhaling, I can be with what is." Once we are clear on the "what is" and centered in how it aligns with our values, we can use our voices to speak up to address it—with compassion and kindness.

Cultivating compassion allows space to act, care, support, and help others intentionally. Practice being compassionate and kind to yourself first, and then do that with others wherever you can. Becoming curious, ask genuine questions, and listen to those around you. It could also look like taking some time to journal to better understand your feelings or reactions, maybe even to notice any reluctance or confusion that is arising. Satya laced with ahimsa allows us to speak up and out about the truths we see and want to create in the world—in ways that others can hear and receive our words. Ishvara pranidhana allows us to commit to taking selfless action for the benefit of all beings.

The writer, performance artist, and online personality Alok Vaid-Menon is an inspiring example of someone who embodies this level of compassion founded in forgiveness. Alok teaches us in so many ways. As a nonbinary trans feminine person, they get many hateful comments on social media. They respond to these comments with compassion and care, seeking to assert their own humanity and, in turn, help commenters see their own as well. They said in a speech in 2022 at Sydney, Australia's Festival of Dangerous Ideas, "I actually don't believe that it's good politics to just blame individuals for prejudice. I have come to understand that the people who harass me, the people who are so obsessed with my appearance, are grieving the gender binary too. I refuse to accept that my life has been reduced to an opinion or to a political belief. We exist, we've always existed. I won't indulge a political discourse that would have me prove that I exist. Instead, I flip the script and say, 'Why do you not accept your own complexity?' Because when you come to accept yourself, you feel no need to police other people."

Alok's artistic expression—poetry, compassion, care, and liberation—and their compassion show us what is possible in the face of dehumanization and hate. Taking any peaceful, productive action is a conscious act of ahimsa. Ahimsa can mean bringing empathy toward ourselves and others, doing whatever we can to stop the harm occurring around us—and the harm pointed at us. Sharing our voices in ways that make the world a better place is a powerful way to practice. There are so many ways to find your voice. You don't need to be perfect, but you can start with clear ahimsa- and satya-aligned actions. Feel your feelings. Acknowledge them. Transform your frustration into poetry or art. Write to your representatives asking for your demands to be listened to and met. Join a march. Donate. Reach out to a friend in need. Take productive, nonviolent action that will help create change.

When we practice interconnection and community care, we remember that our survival and liberation are bound together with the survival and liberation of others. We live to create non-harm for others as well as for ourselves. We practice community care as self-care *with empathy* so that people know they are not alone. We are here together and yoga is supporting us.

The yoga we commit to as agents of spiritual possibility is different from the colonized version most Westerners are used to. Yoga as sadhana comes out of a developmental or competency framework. Ever since the British invaded and colonized India, ever since Westerners have co-opted yoga as their own, it has been misinterpreted—particularly in the West—as achievement oriented.

An achievement model is one that measures your progress based on what you've accomplished—and how well you accomplished it. It's what leads people to say, "I'll never be good at yoga, I can't even touch my toes"; or "I'm not flexible enough." This model leads us to believe that there's only one "fullest expression of the pose." It's also what leads us to say, "Okay, I've mastered these 'advanced' poses and now I'm a yogi."

A developmental or competency model of yoga, on the other hand, is based on *process*, not outcomes. It gives you a clear path to follow to personally grow and deepen. It allows you to develop skills that are connected to areas of growth and practice that align with what it means to live your yoga. There's no "one and done"; no certificate at the end. Rather, it is an ongoing investigation into who you are and how you see your place in the world. The Bhagavad Gita provides a good example of this kind of interior investigation. In the text, Krishna enjoins Arjuna to act out of faith and duty and not let his emotions rule his decisions. Although he reminds Arjuna that the choices he makes will determine his fate (karma), Krishna never tells Arjuna what to do or how to do it. He encourages him to develop a sense of equanimity and to serve without being attached to the results.

According to the *Yoga Vashistha*, an influential sixth-century C.E. spiritual text containing elements of Hinduism and all the Shramanic traditions, even if we have known the truth, we must continue to practice it. From this developmental perspective, once we say yes to the call of yoga, we become agents of spiritual possibility working with yoga as our *theory* of change. Having a yogic theory of change means you have beliefs, ideas, practices, and teachings within the yoga tradition that become a part of how you understand yourself, your relationships, and social systems and how you can help make the world a better place. Your relationship with yoga and your personal theory of change aren't static; they are ever evolving. As we see in the next chapter, it often depends on what stage of life you're in, the obligations you have, and the commitment you are willing and able to make as a spiritual changemaker.

SADHAKAS SPEAK: ANGIE TIWARI
::

My sadhana looks like applying yoga to every single aspect of my life. It's about bringing in the awareness to understand myself better and to understand my relationships more clearly. That includes my relationship with people, work, food, technology, exercise, and more. My self-practice, including deep self-inquiry, has given me so much more clarity than before and has allowed me to put things into perspective. It's also been incredibly helpful when identifying what I want to change in my life and being able to go ahead and do so confidently. When I feel anxious or overwhelmed, I understand myself well enough to know how to self-regulate, and I have my sadhana to thank for this. I also feel more in tune with those around me, more self-aware and connected. This is a lifelong practice and one that I'm constantly growing in and learning from. None of us are perfect, and I believe a dedication to my own sadhana has helped me to stay on track in life, to remain humble and open to constant learning.

—Angie Tiwari, yoga, meditation, breathwork
coach and Ayurveda consultant

7

The Four Stages of Sadhana

Know your duty and do it without hesitation.
—BHAGAVAD GITA

THE DEVELOPMENTAL MODEL of yoga reminds us that there have always been multiple ways to practice yoga or to serve from a yogic heart and mindset. So much depends on where we are in our lives (our ashrama, or stage of life) and what path we've chosen to follow (our dharma). The stages of the developmental model of yoga are really intended to be iterative and descriptive rather than prescriptive. They give us insight into what might be opening up—or conversely, what blocks might be arising—for us at certain stages of practice. These stages are a part of traditional Vedic teachings and are fourfold: they include the life of a student (*brahmachari*); the life of a householder (*grihastha*), the life of a forest dweller or retiree (*vanaprastha*), and the life of a renunciate (*sannyasin*); they guide us as we aim toward developing our highest potential for the greatest good. Every stage has something to offer us in our personal practice, in our relationships, and our work toward justice—in ways that make sense for who we are, our life circumstances, and our personal *svadharma* (self-purpose).

In part 1, I talked briefly about the violent and heinous way the Brahminical patriarchy has appropriated yoga as a means of control and oppression leveled against Dalit folks. Among the many ways those oppressors sought control was by exploiting the concepts of ashramas and dharma. By setting the social order and respective

duties based on caste, gender, and stage of life, the patriarchy jus-
tified and solidified their power. As practitioners of yoga honoring
and embracing its roots today, we must work to upend that and
return yoga to what we believe is the true nature and intention of
these concepts. We must choose the understanding that in every
stage of life, each one of us has something unique to offer the world.
That the true spirit of yoga—based on ahimsa, satya (the soul's truth)
and ishvara pranidhana—has something uniquely personal and
important to offer each one of us regardless of who we are, what we
were born into, or our current circumstances.

BRAHMACHARIN—STUDENTSHIP

As brahmachari, we are learning what it means to live the yogic way.
We are studying—under the tutelage of a teacher—how to live simply, follow the ethical principles of yoga (yamas and niyamas), study
the sacred texts (svadhyaya), and have a practice that is centered on
devotion (ishvara pranidhana). For a brahmacharin, leadership may
mean getting to know yourself as a sadhaka, trying on new ways of
being, or apprenticing with someone whose service in the world
appeals to you.

The brahmacharyin stage begins in childhood, at the advent of
self-discovery, and traditionally ends around age twenty-five. Historically students were young boys and their dedication to their
teacher—their guru—was a step along the path toward adulthood.
For some, this path ended in marriage and a family. For others, the
brahmacharin stage was preparation for further study or for the
monkhood. These days, it is not confined to young boys and their
gurus. Anyone can be in the brahmacharin stage. And many of us
are, as we explore again and again what it means to show up for
justice; what it means to be humble and learn from those who have
more experience or who have lived lives different from our own. No
matter our age or stature, we can humbly take our seat in this stage
of studentship as we seek to be allies and accomplices to others. We
can listen, learn, and do our homework as devoted students of this
sacred practice of yoga. We can also spend time inquiring and fig-

uring out where and how we want to support others. Think about a young child always asking questions of parents, teachers, older siblings—anyone who'll listen—as they discover what it means to get along and share with others, tell the truth, and be generous. What I've discovered in parenting a kid who is at this stage of inquiry is that sometimes they show *me* the way. They share their interpretation of the yogic path, proving that no one is ever too old to be the student.

As a parent and teacher, I was also the student during an afternoon when I taught yoga in my kiddo Kailash's preschool class. I had just finished telling a story about two characters, Penguin and Pinecone, and the way they care for each other,[1] sharing it as an example of practicing ahimsa—love. As we walked outside, another student ran up, punched, and bit Kailash completely out of the blue. Kailash, who was four years old at the time, didn't retaliate. I was activated, though, and asked, "Why didn't you hit back?"

"Because he struggles and I know that. I wanted to help him. It's the power of ahimsa, Mom," Kailash said, "the power of love." Of course. Young kids understand the lessons so deeply. Kailash was certainly my yoga teacher that day.

Brahmacharin Challenges

If this is the stage you're in, know that as you mature, sometimes challenges emerge. For example, beware of an impatient ego. Try not to get ahead of yourself. It can be tempting to think you've got this already, that you know everything you need to know. You don't. Be patient. Keep learning. It's important to stay humble, curious, and empty so that you can receive the wise counsel of your teachers. If your mind is already full of what you think you know, your own experiences and opinions, there is no room for anything else. Empty your mind and receive the teachings.

Another example of a challenge: beware of a crisis of confidence —the old imposter syndrome. *I'm just a student—who am I to think I can live my sadhana? That I can contribute in any meaningful way? How will I ever know enough or be enough?* This can feel so deflating and sometimes even paralyzing. But you don't *need* to know right now. This is the stage of self-discovery in which you get to try things out to see what resonates with you; to discover what you're good at and how you want to get involved. You don't have to be an expert or know everything. That's the beauty of this stage. The more you learn, the more confident you'll become.

⁘ BRAHMACHARIN INQUIRY

* Who are your mentors?
* Who can you turn to for guidance and advice?
* What gets in your way of receiving wise counsel?
* What do you hunger for or desire to learn?
* What does your heart and your practice point you to?   ⁘

GRIHASTHA—HOUSEHOLDER

Grihastha (householder) is the stage of life in which we engage in the world. It is a very creative, active time—we are outwardly directed, making our mark in the world, possibly raising a family, starting new projects, eager and ready to connect with others and share our gifts. We understand ourselves and our practice in relationship to others—family, work, and community. A powerful expression of creative energy surges through us; tapas, or action, becomes our primary focus and fuels our desire to serve others. Whereas the brahmacharin's main investigation focuses on "Who am I?," the grihastha's asks, "What am I? What is my purpose in life?" Our goal is to pursue a virtuous life as well as create enough wealth and resources to sustain ourselves and others in various stages of life. It's important to explore and understand our creative dharma— our purpose in life during this time—as we choose *how* to make money and build a life with our creative energy. Our leadership as a grihastha is often one of doing and acting in the world, ideally informed by the wise counsel of our self-knowledge as well as the spiritual teachers and wise friends we've connected with while in the student stage.

There's a lot going on in a householder's life. This is when we

can—and we must—put our practice to the test as sadhakas. Bringing our spiritual practice into our familial relationships, work, communities, and even our casual interactions as we move through our
day is our duty now. This is when we create connections, clarify our
life purpose, and figure out how best to use our gifts. My own sadhaka path and my commitment to yoga ethics were instrumental in
my decision to choose a loving partner and ultimately start a family.

When Eran and I first met, we bonded over the fact that we were
both considering ordaining into renunciate spiritual traditions. Each
of us had a deep calling to spiritual growth. We kept inviting each
other to silent retreat after silent retreat, spiritual teachings after
spiritual teachings, until we finally realized there was more chem-
istry than just our fire for spirit! We decided we wanted to have a
relationship within a "householder's life," but one founded on yoga
ethics. This way of relating allowed us to really go deep and build
a relationship that has led to twenty years of love and support. As
someone who never thought I'd have a life partner or a child, I surprised myself by growing into a relationship that complements my
freedom rather than constricts it.

Throughout the years we've supported each other's growth—
physically, mentally, emotionally, spiritually. For example, when
I met Eran, he was a wonderful gardener with an almost intuitive
connection to the land. So I encouraged him to expand on his talents
and see where they would take him. As he investigated the many
ways he could do that, and I supported us with my teacher's salary,
he went back to school and studied to become a landscape architect.
He then got to work with some of the biggest themed entertainment
companies designing beautiful outdoor spaces.

It wasn't that long afterward that he reciprocated. As my teaching job ended, Eran supported me as I birthed my social enterprise
business, which became Ignite Institute for Yogic Leadership and
Social Change. Back then, we had very few resources to draw on
and yet he encouraged me to trust myself, do what I loved, and create yoga teacher trainings, something my spiritual teacher in India
had asked me to do. "I'd bet on anything you do," Eran told me as we
took our meager savings and invested it in my very first business.

And it worked! The Ignite Institute for Yogic Leadership and Social Change has trained thousands of students and hundreds of thousands have taken part in our free education and trainings. From the foundation, we keep growing and innovating. Together, we created a wellness-tech project called the Yoke Yoga app. It is a social benefit project to share yoga for anyone who can benefit from it, for free. It centers diverse yoga teachers who bring free yoga to folks who have everyday problems yoga can address. What a gift to have a relationship based on mutual trust, faith, and uplift—built solidly on yogic principles—that allows each of us to grow and go further in our lives together in service and individually.

Our commitment to each other through our spiritual practice has also informed our parenting. Both of us believe it is our dharma to support the next generation and to model what it means to live in a yogic way. As such, I learned early on to regard Kailash not as *my* child or *our* child but as a young being whom I am lovingly tasked with stewarding and helping to grow into their fullest expression. This practice of aparigraha, nonattachment, changes everything! When Kailash does something that frustrates me, I pause for a few breaths, which helps me to not get reactive. And then I remind myself that Kailash is their own soul having their own experience and with their own karma in this world. I do my best to give them guidance but ultimately the path they are on is theirs.

Conscious Parenting

Our responsibility as grihastha parents is to help our children develop tools and skills to connect with themselves and others in a loving, harmonious way. We can provide practices that help them regulate their emotions and that support them on their own yogic path. Simultaneously, as parents, we get to work on ourselves as well.

As a parent, ask yourself: *How is parenting exposing my triggers? What practices can support me? How can I show up in a loving, truthful manner even when my child is behaving in a way that activates me?* You may want to ask yourself, *Is this a cry for help or love?*

When your child gets upset, observe them and then communicate what you noticed: "I can see you're upset. Your body is crunched up, your face is scrunched, and your eyes are down. It's okay. Big feelings are natural and normal." This can help them learn to switch from ignorance of their emotional state to awareness, self-regulate, and begin to manage their own mood shifting. It can also reassure them that you're not judging their emotions or reactions. When in doubt, simply ask, "Do you want to be helped, heard, or hugged?"

Invite your child to practice feeling their emotions. Start by saying, "You had some really big emotions today, didn't you? Tell me about them. Were they a level 2, 3, or 3 billion? What do you think got in the way of you feeling okay? Take some deep breaths and stretch. Yoga helps us regulate our emotions and get to harmony states. Feelings are natural and normal. We get to learn and grow!"

Grihastha Challenges

When you're committed to the yogic path of service, the grihastha stage can pose some unique challenges on personal, relational, and communal levels. How do you manage your time and prioritize your personal practice? The necessary outward-directed focus of the householder can sometimes make it difficult to move beyond what feels immediate—providing for your family and meeting your work commitments—and toward an inward-focused investigation. It can be tempting to forgo your meditation and asana practice because there's so much that demands your attention. What happens when you do that, of course, is you not only run the risk of burning out but you also get further away from knowing yourself—from svadhyaya. What to do? Slow down. Don't be too hard on yourself. Set reasonable boundaries. Start by recommitting to your personal practice in small ways, centering dharana and dhyana to help focus your mind, and gradually build from there until you feel you can meet your grihastha demands with equanimity.

Another challenge householders struggle with is how hard it can be to pay attention to what needs to be done out in the world— beyond the confines of home and work responsibilities. We want to be present with friends, causes, children, elders—but we barely have enough time to do the grocery shopping or fold the laundry. It's so easy to get caught in a kind of attention attrition that happens when living under global capitalism. Who has time (or even the energy) to pay attention to the inequities in our world when everything conspires to keep us busy and our minds scattered? When our time, resources, and energy are so limited? One question I hear a lot is "How can I direct my attention so that it gives the most benefit?" As a grihastha, it helps to remember that there are myriad ways to show up. Look at what you're already doing, where your attention is focused. Sometimes the most important way to serve is to empower the next generation; to model and instill in your children, nieces, and nephews, niblings, or young students the importance of embracing the tenets of samanya dharma, moral or ethical codes that apply to everyone, such as compassionate action; patience; self-knowledge; dedication to justice, truth, and equanimity.

Service in the grihastha stage can look like caring for our communities or the family down the street; being a mindful colleague or thoughtful worker in the office and in your community. It's part of how you fulfill your dharma and show up in your life. In this way, you are participating in creating a more equitable and just future.

⠿ GRIHASTHA INQUIRY

• What is driving you and what are you identifying with right now?

- What is your relationship to your identity? As a partner, a parent, or a creative? How does your identity connect to your dharma?
- What is your gift of service? How do you show up in the world in a meaningful way?
- What's the difference between wanting to help someone and offering your gift of service?
- Are your actions based on true generosity and a desire to make a difference or more on the *appearance* of being generous and what other people will think of you?

VANAPRASTHA—FOREST DWELLER

Although vanaprastha is often referred to as the time of the forest dweller—when the head of the household literally packs up and moves out—leaving home and heading into the woods is not required. For most of us, it means slowing down, simplifying our lives, or often retiring from our jobs. The practice of pratyahara takes center stage here as we begin to let go of worldly attachments—with love and deep respect—and prepare to move toward a more contemplative life. For some, this could mean centering on their meditation practice and spending more time in prayer, in nature, or on retreat. Traditionally, men (it was almost always men) really *did* move to the forest (*prastha*, "moving to"; *vana*, "forest"), leaving their wives and children behind. These days, being a forest dweller means that you relinquish your starring role as householder to the next generation and focus more deeply on your personal sadhana practice. You are no longer responsible for the day-to-day decision-making; you've now taken on a more advisory or mentor role. You've become an elder or an ancestor-in-training. Forest dwellers, by the time they reach this stage, often have a clearer understanding of their dharmic purpose and have expressed it in different ways in service to others.

I sometimes think of vanaprastha as the grandparent stage. So many grandparents I know—including my own parents—tell me that they have a completely different relationship with their grandkids than they did with their own children. They have, in essence, graduated from having to manage the necessities of a kid's life—scheduling, homework, discipline, mealtimes, and bedtimes—and have taken on an adjunct role in the family. I think of them as the *lila* component of family life—playful and creative. They have a sense of freedom that parents don't always have. Grandparents, who are in the vanaprastha stage, are no longer caught up in their obligations at work or even in the home—cooking, cleaning, laundry; they can be more patient and leisurely in their connection with kids. And having lived life for as long as they have, grandparents can be a source of wise counsel, amazing stories, life lessons, and often . . . unconditional love.

Vanaprastha is not a stage specifically for people who have grandchildren—or even children, for that matter. You can play a vital role in young people's lives whether you're a grandparent, an elder relative, a retired friend of the family—as someone who is at least a generation removed from them.

This was clearly illustrated when I was walking with three generations—my father, my child, and myself—to get dinner at a local restaurant. The traffic light opposite the restaurant was counting down from twenty and I sped up to try to cross the road, holding my kiddo's hand tightly. "Oh, at this stage of life, I don't rush to cross the street anymore," my father casually said, dropping some profound wisdom on us. Of course—slow down; focus on the process, the journey and not the destination. What a deep teaching we got that day!

Serving from this stage means cultivating and acting from love; being intentional about the way you show up; serving without being attached to an outcome; and dedicating the merits of such service to the divine. This is ishvara pranidhana played out in real time.

Vanaprastha Challenges

It can be tricky to move from a full life of work and family responsibilities to a quieter, more contemplative stage. It can be hard to know how to let go or to know what to do with yourself; to remember it's no longer your job to involve yourself in the day-to-day. It can be hard to leave the world you've known as you get older. To not find yourself stuck in habits, patterns, and ways of doing things that no longer serve you in this new stage. This is a real opportunity to practice aparigraha, let go, and show up in presence to what is before you. Understandably you may feel you're becoming irrelevant, not needed. Instead of thinking you've *lost* your place, consider that you've *gained* a new role, one in which you can share your wisdom and still have the time to move deeper into spiritual inquiry. It helps to plan ahead for this stage; to engage your family and set some intentions and boundaries that will be beneficial for everyone.

Loneliness is another challenge for some forest dwellers, especially at first, as they move away from the pull of their old life and settle into contemplation. With fewer external distractions, you may find you're questioning who you thought you were and maybe even wondering if you're truly ready for such an inward journey. Don't worry. If this is the path you are walking, it gets easier. Transitioning into the forest-dweller stage can be a gradual thing. You might begin by cutting back on the externals and prioritizing your inner work then move into a mentoring role for the brahmacharins in your life.

⁘ Vanaprastha Inquiry

* What are you beginning to let go of? And, with gentle compassion, how is that letting go going for you?
* What is the hardest part of moving into the forest-dweller stage? The best part?
* What wisdom is arising and becoming born within you?
* What does it mean to move into the mentorship role? What do you feel your role is now in terms of furthering social justice—personally, interpersonally, or socially? ⁘

Sannyasin—Renunciate

The sannyasin stage is marked by a focus on spiritual pursuits of peace and simplicity. The Sanskrit word *sannyasin* literally translates to "throw down" and symbolizes the practice of deeply detaching from material things that bind us to the world. The sannyasin or renunciate stage is different from the vanaprastha stage in that you are no longer preparing or beginning to release your attachments; you've already detached, and your focus is now fully on spiritual growth and connection. Although as a sannyasin you give up any worldly pursuits, you don't reject the world altogether. Instead, your dharma is to share your spiritual wisdom without needing to insist upon it. One can experience this stage at different times in life. What demarcates it is a devotion to the divine and spiritual pursuits above all else. Many Vedic texts, including the Bhagavad Gita, give guidance toward this stage. In *shloka* (verse) 5.3, "One who neither hates nor desires the fruits of his activities is renounced. Such a person, free from all dualities, overcomes material control and is completely liberated."

In the sannyasin stage, the practices of the yamas and niyamas take on even more significance. Nonviolence, nonattachment, and deep devotion to spiritual pursuits are the focus of life. Everything becomes sadhana. The experience of more and more moments of freedom and liberation is a marker of this stage, though these moments can be found throughout all stages of growth and development.

Sannyasin Challenges

In the sannyasin stage, you might notice changes in your body, mind, and vigor. The ways you're used to relating to yourself and the world are shifting. As a sannyasin, you might also face the challenges of ageism, which can be hurtful. Elders can be easily forgotten in our culture or seen as irrelevant, which is a pity because sannyasins are living wisdom traditions in their own right; their intergenerational wisdom is of benefit to everyone. Many younger folks often miss the wisdom and depth of those in this stage. They're too focused on material possessions or too attached to spiritual realizations, and they miss the simplicity and elegance of a sannyasin who resides within this state of moksha—liberation—more and more. There is much to be learned from a sannyasin, but we need to be present in order to do so. We need to learn how to listen.

Two of my main teachers, Shankarji and Thich Nhat Hanh, were in the sannyasin stage when I first met them. I could clearly feel the depth and embodiment of their wisdom teachings. I also noted that though they gave teachings very freely, they weren't trying to convince or force their wisdom on anyone else. They simply were within their wisdom, and those who wished to could come and learn.

Sannyasins have a deep spiritual connection, one steeped in *lived* wisdom. As they renounce material desires and detach from things of the world, their leadership paradoxically becomes more focused and more present. Their detachment can easily be confused with disinterest because it runs counter to our modern, fast-paced, capitalistic society. Yet for folks in this stage, there's nothing that can distract them from their connection to the divine—or dampen their willingness to share their wisdom so freely. It is hard to find examples of folks within this stage, because they are less in the public eye, which makes them even more precious.

⁚⁚ Sannyasin Inquiry

- What supports me in being more present?
- Where is my spiritual practice calling me now?
- Who are my spiritual elders? What can they teach me about showing up and serving in love?
- As a spiritual elder yourself, what do you feel called to share with others?   ⁚⁚

Understanding the ashramas can be very helpful for leading with a spiritual foundation. If you are like me, living, teaching, and writing in the West, where there is less understanding and far fewer structures to support your personal evolution, how do you engage with what makes sense and leave what doesn't serve you? These stages can guide us and bring a sense of connection and humility as we traverse the path to our own spiritual evolution and growth.

It is important to keep in mind, however, that your leadership can progress through the ashramas in a sequential way—associated with your chronological age—and directly connected to the present-moment experience you are having. You can also move around the stages nonsequentially and even experientially—not necessarily attached to age but rather where you are in your life. For example, even at an older age you could be in brahmacharin, the student, stage because of a desire to keep learning, asking questions, and calling in new teachers. Or you may be in the sannyasin, or renunciate, stage in your twenties, feeling the need to withdraw from the world—even for a while—or deciding to live in an intentional or spiritual community. Let the inquiries center you in the stages and experiences you are in, without attaching too much to how old you are, while also bringing awareness that your age may impact your experiences too! It can be both/and.

The Vedic and Yogic traditions understand that people may be in various stages of development. So a brahmacharin, for example, does not need to mock or insult a vanaprasthi but instead understand that there are many ways to practice. That leadership will look different during different times of our lives and should be honored rather than criticized or torn down. A sense that we are all moving in the same direction on the pathway to personal and collective liberation is incredibly helpful. A large dose of humility, compassion, and understanding is the mark of practice at any stage.

No matter which stage of life we're in, as yoga sadhakas we have our duties and purpose to fulfill as we grow, as well as a commitment to use wisdom and the gifts we've been given through our practices to help alleviate the suffering of others. In the next several chapters, I offer a series of eight steps along what I call the sadhakas path that have helped me choose yoga as the lens through which I view the world. In creating the Sadhaka's path, I was inspired by the twelve steps the hero takes in their quest to slay their demons and return victorious and transformed in Joseph Campbell's *The Hero's Journey*. The steps along the path further emerged from the *Hatha Yoga Pradipika*, which offers the keys to unlock the spiritual gate to self-realization as we practice yoga. As in all things yoga, these steps aren't prescriptive; and the path meanders, with no guaranteed straight line to samadhi. Each step offers a descriptive set of skills, tools, and practices you can use to move further inward, connect to the divine within so you can recognize the divine in others, and ultimately do your work in the world from a spiritual and practical perspective.

SADHAKAS SPEAK: DR. GAIL PARKER
⁑

They say you teach the thing you most need to learn. In my case, that's being still, pausing, taking a deep breath or more before I take action. This practice keeps me from acting impulsively. Before I take action, I've learned to let the emotion pass, and then if it still seems like a good idea to do so, I take action. Nine times out of ten, I'm always glad I waited. Along with the emotional readiness to receive whatever the universe is offering, the willingness to be fully present moment to moment, and to remain centered in my own awareness of who I am, the practice of patience is my most profound sadhana practice. My intention is to live a conscious life, and the mindful practice of patience supports my intention. I'm not running a perfect game—no one is—but the daily practice of stillness allows me to check in with myself so that I know the difference between intuition and emotion. They are not the same.

In order to be prepared for whatever comes my way, and to avoid being emotionally hijacked by upsetting events, I listen to my inner intuitive guidance, my wisdom voice. It never fails me.

—Gail Parker, PhD, C-IAYT, psychologist, author

8

Embracing the Call to Yoga

Step 1

Yoga atha anushasanam. *Yoga is now.*
—YOGA SUTRA

THE JOURNEY BEGINS with a call to yoga. We may hear and heed the call several times in our lifetime, and yet it can be fresh and powerful every time. This call to yoga invites us to go deeper into self, relationships, teachings, and action. Some embark on this exploratory journey as adventurers called to the path fully aware and open to its excitements and risks. Some come reluctantly, sensing there's something more to life, but dabble cautiously in growth and transformation. Others come because they've tasted the bliss on their mat and they know there's something more than asana. Still others come through suffering, boredom, wanting more, deep dissatisfaction, a hope for peace and joy, or because they are ready to disconnect from the outer trappings of life such as fame, money, and sensual pleasures, which don't bring lasting peace. However you've arrived, you are here. You've stood at the doorway and crossed the threshold, feeling called to something more. This is the call to yoga.

This call may come in various ways and even at different times in your life. For me, I can locate several distinct calls. As I share my journey, look to find your own in the lines of these stories. See where you find connections and similarities or deep differences that illuminate your own call and journey forward into your story with yoga.

I was born to an Indian father and British mother at a time when interracial marriage was not common. They had looked for months, throughout the English countryside, but no priest or pastor would marry them. Eventually they found one man who could look past prejudice and they wed. Although my family was loving, the world I was born into showed me at every turn I was not wanted. From the housing and workplace discrimination our family endured, to firebombs thrown into Indian and Pakistani families' homes in our neighborhood, to names called out to my brother and me on the playground, to the sneers and nasty looks my family endured as we walked down the road, the messages were loud and clear: *You don't belong here. You are not welcome.* I internalized most of these messages of separation and exclusion without understanding where they came from. I felt insecure, shy, and unworthy of existing. Of course, I did—because that was what I was being told every day by the shopkeepers and the neighborhood bullies in both the UK and later in the US.

Despite everything, because of my family's love and constancy, I always felt safe and wholly me whenever I was in nature. Even at three and four years old, I felt connected to the beauty all around me, and, with no words to describe it, I knew I was in the presence of something sacred, something much bigger than my little self. I had awakened to the joys of sensation—the smells, sights, feels, and tastes of the natural world—and could forget the cruelty of human indignities for a little while. Many times, especially as I got a little older, I experienced moments of transcendent interconnection, a sense of being at one with everything. Looking back at those times, I recognize my connection to the divine as my response to the call of yoga.

Under the duress of great racial tension and violence, with British boys shoving Molotov cocktail explosives into the homes of the few Indian, Pakistani, and mixed families in our region, my family immigrated to the United States in search of a life free from discrimination and full of possibility.

I was four and a half years old when we landed in the San Fernando Valley, a suburb of Los Angeles. We found the possibility, but the discrimination continued. Instead of fighting little British boys, I was fighting American boys, and as we got older, they got bigger and bigger. The gap between a simple, innocent childhood and living under immense racial discrimination widened. There was never a time when I wasn't aware of being treated differently for who I was.

This time, the call to yoga came as an answer to the violence of bullying and discrimination I was enduring all through my childhood. It came through our tradition and my family's practices, which were all about love, safety, and inclusiveness. But I already had such deep training in separation—the opposite of yoga (*yuj*, "union")—that I failed to heed the call. By then, the separation had entered my heart and left me with feelings of inadequacy and unworthiness and made me question why I was even alive.

We tend to think that we are the only ones who have it bad, who feel we don't belong or aren't welcome as we are. But that's not the case. The reasons and the details may differ, but the pain cuts through those differences. You may have had your own version of these experiences. For me, separation showed me all that was missing in my life and reminded me of all that I was not. Of course, I didn't understand that then. The meaning-making of this time didn't happen until much later.

Recognizing the Call

Up in the loft that I shared with my roommate, I could hear everything that happened in the chapel converted to a house. It was hard to sleep and almost impossible to study, but the parties were amazing! I was at University of California, Berkeley, studying philosophy, which demanded intense periods of focus and analysis—nearly impossible with five often-boisterous roommates. I was under an intense amount of stress, and midway through my second year I began to have panic attacks. I found it difficult to breathe and to connect to my breath and body. Unfortunately, I had either forgotten or buried many of the early yogic practices my family had shared with me. The union yoga had given me in my earlier years had been replaced by a sense of complete disconnection between my body, mind, and heart.

I felt trapped and anxious all the time. I knew something needed to shift. One weekend, after a particularly hard night, I found my way to a yoga class at the local YMCA. It was one of those classes with a gem of a teacher who unassumingly and oh-so inclusively guided the class to do what we needed, without pressure or demand. So much of the essence of yoga was present in that room. As we moved, the teacher invited us to stay still in *balasana*, child's pose, if we wished, foreheads pressed into the mat and knees folded under our bodies. I stayed there, tears falling down my cheeks onto the borrowed mat. These weren't tears of sadness, however. They were tears of homecoming and gratitude. This was the call to yoga I needed. And this time I listened. In that peaceful moment of connection between body, mind, and heart, I saw a way out of my anxiety—a way into healing and peace—and that way was through something I'd worked to cut off and reject to fit in. That way was through my ancestral practices, the opposite of separation, an invitation to peace through yoga.

After reading my story, take a moment to think back on your own experiences. Perhaps you've had a similar call into your sense of purpose that helped soften or lift feelings of separation and rejection from the world around you and within you. Perhaps you are clear on your relationship to this ancient practice, even if parts of it remain a mystery to you. However you understand it, you may have also experienced moments of union or reunion through various practices of breath, body, or meditation. Your call to yoga may be simple and mundane or powerful and profound. You may have had multiple calls to yoga that move in spirals or a single one that caught you and held you in its embrace. As the Yoga Sutras teach us, now, in every moment, is a chance to practice yoga. Accepting your call is the first step to deepen your practice and turn toward yoga as a spiritual journey.

⠘ YOGA INQUIRY PRACTICE

* Think back on a time when you experienced the call to yoga. Through joy or suffering or something else. What did that feel like? How did you answer? Tell your story.

- What does the yogic way look like and feel like for you? Describe it in words, images, or collage.
- Create an image of what it means to you to be a vessel for yoga. Paint, draw, collage, journal, sculpt, dance, or play this vessel unique to your experience.   ⁝⁝

Answering the Call

The peace and sense of reconnection I experienced as I accepted the call to yoga aren't necessarily a given for everyone. While it's true that yoga can be uplifting for individuals and populations, others may experience the opposite effect. Like any tool, yoga can be used to heal or harm. Saying yes to the call requires that you learn about and view this ancient practice from the perspective of those who have been harmed and, depending on your social location and positionality—your history, upbringing, culture, and circumstances—from the perspective of *being* harmed. What this means is your relationship with yoga may look very different as a South Asian growing up in India than a new seeker living in the United States.[1] We all must do our part to decolonize the practice—work to untangle the ancient roots of yoga from the misrepresentations heaped upon it by dominant culture—in Western culture as well as within the Brahminical patriarchy. From there, we can begin to investigate what it means to serve in a way that can mitigate and ultimately help reverse the harm yoga has inflicted throughout its complex history and into the present day.

Inner Decolonization

The investigation begins by decolonizing the practice from within. In other words, taking stock of what you have internalized about yoga—what you've been taught, the aspects of the practice you do and don't identify with, what myths you've bought into personally—and noticing how all of that affects you. Colonized yoga is a means to an end—a method of *achieving* something, often under false pretenses. As we discuss in chapter 10, Western yoga's idea of achievement has long been wrapped in a patriarchal archetype of "success": a strong, flexible, thin, and able body that performs certain postures and looks like a paragon of good health. Under the Brahminical patriarchy in colonized India, yoga was appropriated to cement their power and achieve dominance over groups of people they deemed inferior and not worthy, and it's important to be aware of how this may continue today.

To decolonize yoga within ourselves, we must let go of the need for yoga to *be* a certain way and make room for how it's showing up in us, which isn't always easy to do. The focus on achievement traps us into believing that we aren't capable enough, smart enough, worthy enough, talented enough—or whatever our personal "not-enoughs" are—to teach or even practice yoga. This lack of confidence can easily spiral into imposter syndrome, a psychological pattern in which a person doubts their skills, talents, or accomplishments and has a persistent internalized fear of being exposed as a "fraud." The person is convinced that nothing they do will ever be good enough.

All of these feelings are part of the human condition, of course. But they are exacerbated by the goal-oriented, achievement-based systemic oppression and subtle/not-so-subtle messages that tell us we've failed; that people in marginalized groups are "inferior" and will never be enough. When we don't see a process-based path that focuses on skills and competencies that we know how to go toward—when we don't see people who look like us doing yoga, meditation, mindfulness, and wellness practices—we can feel very discouraged and disheartened.

Sometimes acknowledging and naming the systemic nature of these exclusions, messages, and internalizations can be a step toward disentangling them from our consciousness—and helping to ensure we aren't contributing toward further oppression. I remind myself that these process-based practices come from people of color seeking their own and others' liberation—and have been practiced by our ancestors for thousands of years. This understanding helps me feel more present and confident in taking up space and encouraging others to do the same. The call to yoga is a call to confront and interrupt these systems and messages that make people feel like yoga is for some and not for all.

The practice of inner decolonization is not a one-and-done exercise. It's something we must revisit repeatedly. Here are some tools I've found helpful on my own path.

1. **Acknowledge** the systemic nature of these blocks. Remind yourself that there may be social conditioning, achievement-based imperatives, oppression, and inequity at play that feed a sense of inner doubt.

2. **Reframe** your thoughts. Beginning something new is rarely easy. That's okay. Know that you'll get better with practice. Don't compare yourself to others or some future state of perfection. Talk back to your inner critic. Remind yourself of all the reasons that you can be of service; all the ways you are interesting and fun; or all the aspects that make you a good friend or yoga teacher right now!

3. **Accept** defeat. True failure—or the feeling of it—often has unique and often important teachings within it. In fact, the times I've failed have been my greatest teachers, but maybe not right away. The gift is often something I need to reflect upon and come to understand on my own. Often the growth we want is on the other side of acceptance—and risk for something more.

4. **Support** the mind, using mantra, such as AUM, or inner affirmations, replacing negative self-talk with positive thoughts: *I am enough just as I am. I am worthy. I am calm.*

5. **Reach out** in advance. Find a community that shares your values in this practice. It can be helpful to have circles, colleagues, friends, or sangha to connect with—people who can support and lift you up and you, in turn, can do the same.

6. **Consider** that the reason you're so anxious or concerned could be because you care so much. Tune in to the feeling and the values below the concern and let those feelings of love nourish and connect you. Practice aparigraha—loosen the grip, let it go. I find it helpful to ask myself: *What's the worst-case scenario? Can I deal with that? Or better still,* how *would I deal with that?*

7. **Practice** self-love, self-care, and self-compassion! Know that

this work can help to heal the past traumas of your ancestors—all those generations who came before you—and stop that intergenerational trauma from being passed on to future generations. It is powerful. You are growing. You are learning. You got this! I remind myself: *Trust that I am the message.* Get out of the way and let the gift come through you. Remember: you are a vehicle for the teachings.

8. **Reconnect** to your practice and offer it up as service for the liberation of all. Don't neglect time on your mat or your cushion, which gives you the opportunity to reflect, recharge your batteries, and recommit to your sadhana. Interrupt oppression within and without.

Decolonization Explores Causes and Conditions of Separation

In a system and context where colonial oppression has taken away agency to practice Indigenous healing and strengthening practices such as mindfulness, meditation, and yoga, we must remember that colonization of yoga is not a metaphor. It's a practice that perpetuates a relationship of exploitation, a system that strips power from some while allowing those who claim power to continue to benefit from stealing natural resources and labor, as well as the ideas and cultural knowledge of Indigenous people.

Colonization causes harm to everyone because oppression harms both the oppressed and the oppressor. For those of us who are Indian or who come from colonized people and places, our familial and spiritual lineages may have been fractured and our wisdom hidden or lost. For those of us whose ancestors were the colonizers, we may have been cut off from our own cultures as well as from our sense of connection, compassion, and humanity. The devastating power of oppression is that it divides us, pitting individuals and groups against one another. It prevents meaningful dialogue and connection with the larger community, and it separates us from our ability to connect with our bodies, minds, and hearts.

To be colonized is to become a stranger in your own land. This is the feeling many Indian people have in most Westernized mindfulness, meditation, embodiment, and yoga spaces today. This colonization happens when the full, complex breadth of Asian traditions' intention for the practice of liberation is reduced to fewer than its many limbs. It happens when yoga is diminished to a practice whose intent is to perfect physical strength or prowess; a practice solely aimed at reducing stress so we can be cogs in a wheel of production and consumption.

Like colonization, decolonization is a process as well as an outcome. It is multilayered and it happens over time. In "Decolonization Is Not a Metaphor," the scholars Eve Tuck and K. Wayne Yang point out that decolonization is specific to repatriation. They use the United States as a prime example, in which the colonists arrived, took over land from Indigenous people, and never left. Their claim is that for decolonization to happen, land must be returned to the Indigenous people from whom it has been stolen.[2]

In our yoga practice, decolonization is also not a metaphor. It is an act of restoring sovereignty, resources, goods, wealth, land, spiritual riches, power, and knowledge. Decolonization means to re-indigenize or create reparations on multiple levels for those most impacted. But decolonization is *not* a way to further fundamentalist claims that yoga is an exclusive Hindu tradition; it is *not* a way to use indigeneity to unseat others from their place within yoga; it is *not* a way to police ourselves or others who practice, insisting that unless you have attained certain benchmarks, you aren't a true yoga practitioner. Decolonization *is* both complex and multilayered. It's the means of reinstating yoga as the path that leads us toward liberation and transcendence; as practices and skills that unite us with the broken or shameful parts of ourselves and with groups we think of as "different" or "other."

Here are a few ways I believe we can begin to decolonize yoga and other practices from South Asia.

1. **Preserve** the language. Learn about the many languages of yoga and meditation, including Sanskrit and Pali. It is important to share language as a community and bring empathy

and authenticity to the words we use. You can work to pro-
nounce words correctly—whether or not you use them in
your teaching or other dharma work. Preserving language is
a powerful means of preserving culture. At the same time, by
understanding the ways Sanskrit has been used to exclude,
you can strive to *include* rather than exclude.

2. **Include** diverse South Asian perspectives, values, and cultural respect in daily practices. Think critically about what
power structures this might be holding up, including awareness of interrupting Brahminical patriarchy. Work to center
liberatory voices. For example, ask diverse South Asian practitioners to share their experiences with a variety of meditation, mindfulness, and yoga practices. Learn from their
Indigenous knowledge—ancient texts, meditation practices,
shlokas, chanting. Tap into their traditional knowledge—all
the inherent and sometimes more esoteric practices of the
tradition: the eight-limbed path; purification rituals; ways to
live a conscious, compassionate life. It is important to include
a variety of perspectives, religious and cultural backgrounds,
and lineages and to include South Asian practitioners who
take radical and nontraditional approaches as well.

3. **Practice** decolonial modes of knowledge and experience.
For example, decolonizing your mindfulness or yoga practice can come through something concrete like the music
you play in an embodiment, meditation, or yoga asana class.
Including music from Indian, Desi, and South Asian musi-
cians and artists can help us learn more about context.

4. **Thoughtfully position** knowledge that comes from the land
and the people and their stories and ways of knowing at the
heart of all that we do. Include cultural practices in the oper-
ations of our schools, studios, and institutions.

5. **Cite** correct cultural references. To do that, explore, learn,
and begin to appreciate the complex culture and history
from which this tradition comes. Commitment to deep practice, questioning, and learning is part of the answer.

6. **Inquire deeply** by engaging with other yoga teachers. Don't shy away from penetrating and sometimes difficult questions to hold ourselves accountable. To do this, bring the whole of yourself to the table. We can name that yoga has been used as a tool to harm as well as to heal. An important question to ask: *For whom is yoga accessible today and how can I address its legacy of past injustices through my teaching practice and my life?*

7. **Embody and share** *all* aspects of yoga and meditation, including all eight limbs of yoga, not just asana. Right now, the West equates meditation with stress reduction and yoga with exercise. The culture of these wisdom traditions is missing. Non-native practitioners and teachers must commit to experiencing and understanding the diversity of yogic culture as it is conveyed through its lineages across the Indian and diasporic culture. There needs to be a thorough and consistent exposure to and an appreciation of culture.

8. **Reinforce** a clear demarcation between appreciation and appropriation through the lens of understanding privilege, dominance, caste, colonization, and supremacy. When we humbly and respectfully consider yoga's history, its context, and its many branches and practices, we give ourselves a fighting chance to achieve yoga's aim of enlightenment of mind, body, and spirit.

9. **Repair.** Reparations are a way of atoning for what has been stolen and returning the benefits, rights, and profits of a culture's inheritance to its creators. Those of us who benefit from the teachings of yoga must give back to the communities from whom this practice has come. Reparations in yoga happen alongside and in conversation with other movements for reparations, such as those for slavery.

10. **Connect** to your own creativity and lineages first before connecting to others.

11. **Honor** and acknowledge the Brown and Black people from whom this practice has come by practicing spiritual lineage acknowledgment. Do this—much like you do a land acknowledgment—at the beginning of any yoga-related class, work-

shop, training, or event, either in person or online. For a deeper exploration of the colonization and decolonization of yoga, read *Embrace Yoga's Roots*.

Decolonizing our learning is a crucial step that prepares us to answer the call to yoga. As we let go of perfectionism and turn away from outward messages and ideals of what something is *supposed* to be, as we reject the use of yoga to divide and oppress, we are free to cross the threshold and commit to yoga as our spiritual practice. It's not always easy to go all in; we'll see in the next chapter all the ways we resist the call—and explore how best to work with our minds and our bodies to step onto the path of service.

WAYS TO OFFER REPARATIONS

##

Reparations within the yoga, meditation, and mindfulness community can look many ways. Here are some suggestions:

- Spend your money on those from whom this practice came.
- Hire diverse South Asian/Desi teachers.
- Hire and consult with BIPOC race equity and yoga teachers.
- Learn and practice the full expanse of what yoga can be.
- Buy books written by diverse South Asian authors offering various perspectives.
- Actively interrupt caste-based oppression and discrimination.
- Donate money to organizations doing humanitarian work in India or organizations dedicated to the preservation of the wisdom, mindfulness, meditation, contemplative, and yoga traditions within India.

9

Choosing a Spiritual Life
Step 2

Only when we pierce through this magic veil do we see the
One who appears as many.
—*SHVETASHVATARA UPANISHAD*

EACH TIME you step on your mat to practice asana; each time you
sit on a cushion and breathe, do pranayama, or meditate; each time
you open a sacred text or show up to serve in love, you are crossing
a threshold to a deeper spiritual commitment. Each time you cross
one of these thresholds, you make the choice to step into your power
and bring the spiritual aspects of yoga that are within you forward in
a deeper way. You embrace the practice in its root intentions before
systems of oppression and domination twisted and shaped it.

Crossing such a threshold involves leaving behind many supportive constructs that you may have outgrown. Your thresholds (and
there are many!) may be crossed not once but thousands of times.
Each time, you must leave the comfortable confines of familiar structures and embark on a journey into the unknown, leaving behind
the belief that you have to be perfect or seen as worthy in some way
in order to turn toward practice. You are already worthy. Always. It
can take remembering that yoga is a mindset, a way of being in the
world that you can touch into at any moment. It can be letting go of
people-pleasing, putting others' needs before your own. It can be
practicing self-forgiveness and self-compassion. Maybe you haven't
made it to your mat or cushion in a day, a week, a month, a year.

Maybe you weren't the kindest or most present parent, friend, partner this week . . . and yet today you show up. It doesn't matter how many steps or decisions you've made that pull you away from center or from your highest intentions; it just takes one decision to come back.

I see students cross a threshold into a deeper spiritual commitment when they sign up for teacher training or a workshop. They often come in with doubts. They wonder if they are worthy or capable, or if the path will work for them. Despite these very human questions, they take the leap and decide to try. The wish to expand, to grow, to learn, to say yes to who they are becoming are all reasons they give for taking this leap. Often crossing the threshold can be simply a matter of choice—a choice to step into one's own power, the power of a container of learning, and a commitment to oneself to embrace yoga as a way of life and service.

There are questions to ponder and new experiences to unpack at the threshold. What are you leaving behind? What are you taking with you? As you say farewell to the person you were and open up to growth and change, you may experience grief. That's normal; take all the time you need to acknowledge and feel it, to mourn what you've left so that you can create room to embrace what's next.

As sadhakas, we must leave behind anything that gets in the way of our commitment to spiritual growth. This can mean making a monumental decision, such as leaving a toxic relationship, moving to a new country, or changing jobs. It can also be little moments of releasing one thing and welcoming or reconnecting with something else. For example, choosing to replace an evening Netflix session with meditation, journaling, self-care, or a conversation with a spiritual friend can be a welcome shift. You get to determine the shifts that will support you in crossing your threshold to deeper spiritual connection.

It took me many years to cross the threshold and turn toward yoga as a way of life. I ran from it for a long time, afraid of the judgments of my peers and family. I needed to decolonize my thinking about yoga as something I was unworthy of, having internalized the judgmental and normative messages of yoga in the West. I needed to decolonize my understanding and return to the original truth of yoga, as shared in yoga philosophy as inclusive and available for everyone. And then finally I made a grand gesture as a way of saying yes to this path: I bought a one-way ticket to India and told myself I wouldn't come back until what I went there for was complete! It was my sankalpa—a promise I made to myself to say yes to my heritage, to listen to the call of my ancestors, and to feel the true meaning of yoga in my bones and heart. As I arrived, I remember breathing deep, knowing that I was home.

Grand gestures can be one way to cross the threshold. But they are not necessary. I cross the threshold every morning when I sit down on my cushion instead of scrolling, each time I offer a compassionate word to myself or a friend, or each time I take a mindful pause to breathe. As my student Leigh Green says, "I remind myself that the only thing yoga requires me to do is breathe. And once I connect my breath and intention with my body, everything else— the shame and overthinking—falls to the wayside. Then I can freely access the joy that I'd been unintentionally withholding from myself for decades."

⠶ CROSSING THE THRESHOLD PRACTICE

- Lay down a stick, string, or even a yoga mat to delineate a "threshold" that, once crossed, solidifies your commitment to practice. Stand on one side of the threshold. Take some time there to reflect on who you are on this side of the threshold. What has brought you here? What do you need to leave behind in order to cross to the other side? Really take your time with this. It may come out as a dance, a cry, movement, journaling, a scream, or a fart. Let it all out.
- Then, when you feel ready—and only you will know when that is—step, leap, dance, or tumble across to the other side of your threshold. Take some deep breaths here. Who are you becoming at this moment? What is here for you in this new way of being and this new place in your life?   ⠶

Meeting Inner Resistance

No matter how many times you cross your symbolic threshold, moments of doubt may crop up. Have you ever noticed that can happen even when you're fully into it? That within the call to adventure and exploration there's also the knock and pull of resistance? This pull is the unwanted visitor on any journey into the soul—and the sadhaka's journey is no exception. It may show up in the voice that says *You aren't ready* or *You don't have a strong practice*, or *You don't deserve to feel this good or peaceful*.

Resisting the call to go deeper with yoga can show up in various and sometimes surprising ways. Though resistance is here as part of step 2, it can be an unwelcome guest any time on the yogic path, no matter how long you've been practicing. The way resistance shows up again and again reminds us that the steps are process-oriented and not at all linear. We can revisit the tools for working with resistance wherever we are on our path. Once we name resistance, we can often defuse its power to sabotage our lives. Here are some of the most common signs of resistance:

I Have No Time

This is a big one for many of us. We may have a life filled with commitments, obligations, and joys. We might work or be in school or both, we may have caregiving commitments, and we all have basic bodily needs such as to eat and sleep. We may feel like there's no time left for self or practice. Sometimes that's indeed the case. However, is it true? For many of us, yoga isn't separate from life. We could make time if we were more strategic or intentional and allowed yoga into every aspect of what we do. So, what's underneath that resistance?

When I became a new mom, I had to learn that my yoga practice might look completely different from one day to the next. Just because I couldn't carve out an hour or more every morning didn't mean I had to give yoga up entirely. During early infancy and toddler time, ten- or fifteen-minute practices—even five minutes!—was enough for me to check in with myself, do a few rounds of pranayama, and reconfirm my commitment. Even doing metta (loving-kindness) meditation while nursing or changing diapers became a deep practice. Parenting became a study in how we can apply our yoga wherever we are.

Notice with patience and kindness your own reluctance to practice. Maybe, like me, you've had a relationship with yoga that must change its form. Maybe you feel that with your busy schedule, you can no longer commit to the sadhaka path in the way you used to. Instead of abandoning your practice completely, get creative. Think of ways to include *moments* of practice instead of hours. What can you do in two minutes? Five minutes? Thirty minutes? Don't get caught up in what should be or what used to be. Consider what is possible in this very moment—and do that.

I Don't Have a Proper Place to Practice

I hear this form of resistance from students and practitioners a lot: "My space is so tiny. There's no place to put down a mat. I have to get organized—everything is such a mess!" It's a very natural urge to think that we have to make the space perfect for our practice. However, that urge can be a distraction from just sitting down or just moving in ways that open what is really under the surface. Not long ago, a few of my students and I were laughing about how there are some days when just about anything can distract from practice. For example, one of them shared, "I get on my mat to practice and the next thing I know, I'm sweeping dust bunnies from under the bed. Wait! Where did my peaceful practice go?" Everyone laughed as they admitted they could relate. This is such a normal form of resistance to depth. In her book *Yoga at Home*, the yoga teacher and holistic healing mentor Linda Sparrowe calls this "the terror of exactitude"— the need to create the perfect environment for practice. Remembering her words reminded us to surrender to the messiness of life, the messiness of practice, and allow even the messiness of our space to reflect that nothing needs to be perfect—not our surroundings, our practice, or ourselves. It is indeed a privilege to have any amount of time and room to practice.

When people tell me they can't practice because they don't have the right clothes, mat, or money to go to a class, I immediately want to reply, *You don't need any of that to do yoga!* Money or scarcity of resources can become an obstacle. There are real material conditions of lack that can prevent folks from accessing practice. Having said that, the beautiful thing about practicing yoga is that you can do it anywhere—by a stream, under a tree, in that little space between your coffee table and couch—anywhere free of bugs, as Iyengar suggests in *Light on Yoga*. And cute outfits are not required.

I've Lost My Confidence

This type of self-imposed resistance surfaces often, as we saw in earlier chapters. Even longtime practitioners and teachers are not immune to crises of confidence. They may be thinking, *Who am I to bring yoga out into the world? What if I'm really appropriating instead of appreciating? What if I have nothing to offer?* This is a common concern that many students voice. So how do you regain your confidence? By recommitting to your practice in a way that moves you into dialogue with your own body, mind, and heart. To do that, I find it helpful to come back to the niyamas, particularly the last three—tapas, svadhyaya, and ishvara pranidhana.

Tapas allows you to burn up any obstacles on your spiritual path and rekindle your passion for practice. It is the willpower, the determination you need to begin again. Integral to being a yoga steward means going inward before you venture outward. That's where the practice of svadhyaya is useful. Svadhaya reminds us not to focus on what's wrong with us or what needs to be fixed but rather to ask, *What is coming in my day? How am I doing? What do I need?* Based on what surfaces, we may do a few minutes of pranayama, read scripture, do a little yoga asana, meditate with a gentle inward attention—or take a nap.

Finally, ishvara pranidhana, often translated as "humility" or "faith," helps us turn toward resistance and invites us to bring the ancient teachings with us onto our mat and cushion and into daily life. By letting go of what we think we have to do and who we think we need to be, and opening to the power of compassionate action, we can offer others the gifts that yoga has given us. Whatever the form our practice—and ultimately our service—takes, it is wonderful the way it is. Imperfectly perfect. It is a way to find silence and connection.

Think of resistance as a momentary pause to reflect, recalibrate, and move into deeper intimacy with yourself and with yoga. Using this practice of turning toward resistance, you can begin to bring yoga into other areas of your life. Once that happens, so many things become "dharma doors" that open to you, inviting you to practice yoga in everything you do—all day long. Listening to a friend who needs support, breaking up an argument, fighting, caring for someone in need, handling a work deadline, speaking with a challenging colleague—these are all dharma doors—all opportunities to practice personal and collective care and show up for yourself and others with compassion. The antidote to resistance is in the power of choice. We can continue to make choices to turn toward practice and, in doing so, we will inevitably go deeper. I thank my resistance when it arises as I have come to recognize it as a sign that I am growing and my practice is about to deepen yet again.

▒ RESISTANCE PRACTICE

Resistance can be a tool of insight. This is one of the most useful and powerful practices I've found for shifting and moving through resistance.

Sit, stand, or lie down in an easeful way. Place your hands on your body in a way that brings comfort. I often place my right hand on my heart and my left hand on top of my right hand, to bring connection to my heart space. Bring any resistance you feel into your heart space, silently name it, feel it bubble up, and then send self-care and self-compassion there. Notice any negative self-talk arising. Investigate what lives under that self-judgment. Don't spend too long here. Just enough to understand the messages you are receiving. Take three deep, releasing breaths.

Based on what you learn, practice active self-compassion. Say, in your mind, *I forgive myself for believing . . .*, and then, *I forgive myself for thinking. . .* And then turn the insight into an affirmation. For example, you might say, *I forgive myself for believing I am unworthy of peace. I forgive myself for thinking that about myself. I affirm that I am worthy of peace.*

End with three deep breaths.   ••
                                                                          ••

SADHAKAS SPEAK: MELISSA SHAH

••

My sadhana is sacred. I wake up every morning to spend time being with my body, mind, and spirit, listening to what they have to tell me. I do the same practice daily, and it changes over time with the support of my mentor/teacher. When I practice, it is an offering to my true self, spirit, the source of inner knowing. Sadhana is meant to be adapted to each individual's physical, mental, and spiritual needs, and there should be a sense of direction as well. Meaning, over time you are moving toward certain practices that will support your goals.

My practice is encased in the breath and guided by it. Every movement is led by the breath and ends with the breath. This has been a powerful practice in my daily life. How can I use my breath to inform my decisions, build a feeling of safety in my body, and develop clarity?

My sadhana is so sacred. Every *uttanasana*, every *surya namaskar*, every pranayama practice, every drop of rest is an offering.

—Melissa Shah, yoga therapist, MPH

FACING CHALLENGES AND CRITICS

The resistance you encounter when committing to the path of practice isn't always internal. In fact, it's not unusual to face conflict and challenges from the outside as well. There may be people who doubt your sincerity, question your motives, and disparage your abilities. Listening to them often fans the flames of self-doubt and can cause you to question your motives. Is it possible to stay the course without being derailed by it all?

It's hard enough that we struggle to believe in ourselves. On top of that, many of us must deal with challenges intrinsic to the culture we live in. The most egregious example of this is when others deem us as too Black, Brown, old, fat, or queer to be taken seriously—and there's very little we can do to counter those limiting beliefs, especially without allyship. This is systemic oppression. The doors slam shut and it becomes almost impossible to interrupt the status quo without completely upending the system that fosters oppression in the first place. Cultures of comparison and competition harm us all. Systemic oppression is harmful for everyone because it holds us to unrealistic norms. How do we change this? We need to name systems, and we need each other. We can't do it alone.

Our external challenges can be anything from these oppressive systems to outside criticism, jealousies, power struggles, and more. If you already suffer from inner resistance and doubt, these external challenges can make it even more difficult for you to get out there and be taken seriously as a teacher or even feel welcome as a practitioner. *What if I don't look like a teacher? Am I even strong enough, flexible enough, or thin enough to step into a yoga studio?* Sometimes physical or emotional challenges occur that legitimately change our lives and the trajectory of our practice. Being a lone voice practicing yoga as service and liberation can feel isolating and lonely in a studio or city where this perspective isn't shared. Naming structures and systems of oppression can help in these circumstances. Or, for example, an injury can change how you think about yourself as a practitioner and teacher. It can prompt achievement-oriented thinking: *What if I can no longer do 108 sun salutations because of my shoulder injury?* Sometimes a challenge can become an ordeal—something that can be ongoing or long term—a breakup of a relationship, the loss of a job, your physical or mental health, or the death of someone close to you.

Perhaps the biggest part of any ordeal is not even the sense of loss or the gaping hole it leaves behind, though of course this can feel immeasurable. Instead, it might be the doubt, self-judgment, lack of worthiness we feel within ourselves, disconnection from ourselves or a higher and greater power, or the betrayal of falling out of trust.

⠿ DEALING WITH CONFLICT THE YOGIC WAY

Yoga helps us get in touch with our emotions so we can self-regulate, solve problems, communicate, and heal. Yoga philosophy sees positive moods and harmony states as our birthright. This five-step process can help us manage our moods and move toward problem-solving.

- **Aware.** Become aware of what you are feeling. Conflict is a sign that something is out of alignment with our values. Bring awareness to what is there, notice and name feelings to understand what you need.
- **Calm.** Take a few moments to calm yourself enough so you can create the space to understand what's happening. Breathe, move your body, or curl into a little blanket-fort burrito for a few minutes! Do whatever works.
- **Switch.** It's possible to regulate your emotions and switch your state of mind. Again, spending time moving, breathing, and practicing can help. Even a few minutes of slow, sweet sun salutations aligned with the breath can do the trick.
- **Engage.** Once you feel calmer, check in with your perceptions, name systemic issues if needed, and make room for other points of view. Notice if it's easier now to clarify the challenge and solve the problem.
- **Surrender.** Let go of past experiences and limiting beliefs. Surrendering conflicts from the past allows us to be present in the moment.

Yogic tools help us be responsible for our own emotions. We can reregulate and harmonize our nervous systems, identify stressors, and transform conflict as we move more into more spiritual, harmonious states.   ⠿

Handling Criticism

How can we approach criticism from the yogic perspective of knowing ourselves as good, whole, and complete? From a foundation of enoughness but not from entitlement? We can remain open to learning and growing. For many people, their biggest fear is being "canceled"—called out publicly, humiliated, shamed, and told they're wrong so vehemently that the whole world (or so it seems) turns to watch and nod, celebrate, sign, or chortle along. This sounds terrible when you think about it. It's like your inner critic has grown larger and louder and has spilled out into the world.

When we commit to anything passionately—I mean, really take it on—in our personal life or the public arena, we open ourselves up to criticism. There will be those who don't like how we do things and those who feel compelled to interrupt, critique, or comment on our every move. There will be those who don't like how we look, how we speak, or what we have to say; those who question our motives and our bona fides. I sometimes think of them as "enemies," not because they're trying to cut off my head with a sword but because in some cases I feel like they are trying to assassinate my character!

How can you work with them without forgetting yoga's basic principles of kindness, compassion, and truth? Obviously, there are many ways to do this. Here are a few I've found helpful. As you read along, imagine you've been criticized, or remember a time when what you said was called into question, either privately or publicly.

Notice, Pause, and Breathe

When a criticism is leveled at me, the first thing I do is recognize that the person reacting is upset and unloading their anger, hurt, frustration, fear, or pain onto me. At that moment, their nervous system has likely become dysregulated. As long as I'm not actually oppressing or harming them, I need to step back and take a pause. Breathe. Notice what's happening in my own body. I ask myself, *How is your breath? Where are you feeling tension in your body? How's your heart? What thoughts are running in your mind?*

Harmonize Your Nervous System

Yogic tools can help move you from disharmony to harmony, or what some call emotional regulation. When anything negative or potentially harmful is directed at you, your nervous system can also become dysregulated, along with your criticizer's. At that point, it is hard for anyone to offer a compassionate or measured response. Before you can even assess what is yours and what is not yours so you can respond in a kind or measured way, you have to discharge the energy from your body. When I'm alone, to start this discharge of energy and harmonize myself, I might get physical—jumping, shouting, wiggling, or shaking—or even throwing an impromptu dance party in my living room. Sometimes, I'll call a friend to vent or talk through the feelings I'm experiencing. (Caveat: Always make sure to check in with your friend first to see if they have space at that moment to listen or help problem-solve.) Other times, I'll get quiet and call on my ancestors or guides, listening for and trusting their counsel to help me let go of fear and surrender to the process. You might try different yogic practices to support you in moving from disharmony to harmony and understanding how to get centered and in alignment with your own truth. Centering in your truth is powerful. From there, it becomes easier to keep what is for you and leave the rest.

Compassion: Look for the Gold in the Criticism

Often, underneath the sting of the words being spoken, when we can put aside our initial reaction, we can find something of value in the criticism. Other times—let's be real—what the critics are saying offers nothing of value; their words are simply meant to hurt you or tear you down—and build themselves up. It's important to see and understand the difference between constructive and destructive criticism. We see a lot of both on social media. When you put yourself out there, you're fair game—haters are going to hate just because they can. Anyone can say anything—and they do! I get this kind of criticism from people who write to me to say, "You are just jealous because your nose looks like this. . ." or "This type of person is the best. You are just bitter because you don't rule."

When people attack you based on what you look like or where you come from—or sling other criticisms that are equally without merit—don't waste your time looking for the gold because there is none. Remember you are not required to respond to or engage with them in any way. They are just being mean and hurtful. Ignore them and move on. I know that's often easier said than done. I often get plenty of "likes" and positive feedback on social media, and yet when I see even one unkind or negative comment in the mix, what do you think happens? My mind immediately fixates on that one unkind remark, which I decide completely nullifies all the other positive ones. I remind myself to let it go, that social media can be extreme and there are certain comments that don't warrant a response.

Having said that, I never want to discount or dismiss helpful feedback from thoughtful critics—even when it stings. I've come to understand criticism as a path of radical belonging and compassion. I want to dig deeper to see where the gold is and where the truth lies. To do that, I often check in with my body to see how it is reacting to such feedback. If I notice contraction, tension, or resistance, that's generally an indication that I need to pay attention to what's being offered because that's where learning and growth can happen if I allow it. Insightful feedback is an incredible gift to receive. It allows me to strengthen and soften into more compassion and understanding of myself and others.

As we leave behind the illusion of separation, guided by these teachings in the Upanishads and yogic practice, when we can remember that all perspectives are welcome, when we can stay open to different points of view (even if we don't agree with them), we will be better able to receive them from a more spacious, humble, and interconnected state—one that resembles what we know to be yoga. At the same time, it's important to be discerning and not let others drain our energy or distract us from our true purpose. Keep going!

⣿ CHALLENGES AND CRITICS PRACTICE

- Think of a time in which you received criticism that really stung. Notice if it still lives in your body—and how it manifests. Is there any value in the criticism? Anything you've learned from it? If so, can you acknowledge it and transform the criticism into a gift? If it's not something that has merit, what can you do to let it go?
- Use the following statement as a prompt for journaling, drawing, painting, or any other creative expression of inquiry: *When fear of criticism creeps into my work, it looks like . . .*
- Is there any place where you are holding back because of fear of criticism?
- How can I tangibly offer myself compassion for my fear and keep moving forward? For example, can I talk to a trusted friend and then continue to take the steps in the direction of my passion and goals?   ⣿

SADHAKAS SPEAK: MICHELLE CASSANDRA JOHNSON
⣿

The practice I will describe here came to me during a moment of crisis. I asked for guidance and practices that would help my nervous system settle and bring me back into a state of calmness. I was moving through a separation from my partner, preparing to move across the country, closing my private social work practice, and beginning a new job. It was a tumultuous time, and this sadhana was what I needed exactly. My sadhana looks like preparing honey-lemon water with honey from my honeybees. Then I prepare my altar by lighting a candle, adding any sacred objects I feel are needed, and setting up my meditation cushion. If my dog, Jasper, is in the room, I will set up his meditation cushion as well. I sit on my cushion and meditate for five to ten minutes, sometimes longer. After sitting for a few minutes, I pray to Spirit, my ancestors, and guides. I pull a divination card from one of my many decks, journal to engage in a practice of self-reflection and study, and write ten gratitude statements. Sometimes I end my practice with a guided meditation focused on self-love and connection. This is my sadhana and has been for over five years now.

—Michelle Cassandra Johnson, MSW, LCSW,
500 RYT, YACEP

10

Honoring Relationships

Step 3

> When perfect friendship exists, either between two hearts
> or within a group of hearts in a spiritual organization, such
> friendship perfects each individual. True friendship unites
> two souls so completely that they reflect the unity of Spirit.
>
> —PARAMAHANSA YOGANANDA,
>
> *HOW TO LOVE AND BE LOVED*

AS OUR PRACTICE BECOMES integral to who we are and how we
approach our daily lives, we begin to see that yoga has always been
about relationships. As sadhakas, our personal practice—indeed, our
commitment to the eight-limbed path—guides us in how we choose,
how we develop, and how we show up in relationships—*all* relationships, throughout our entire life, including the relationship we have
with ourselves. In fact, in the forest dweller/renunciate stage, practitioners discover that the key to spiritual development lies in how
they interacted with one another and in their communities *before*
choosing a life of contemplation. In the student and householder
stages, yoga is a profoundly practical tool along the sadhaka path
that helps us employ discernment and equanimity as we enter and
navigate friendships; as we connect with coworkers, casual acquaintances, and our larger community. It informs how we show up with
our kids and in our love relationships; how we choose collaborators and even (and sometimes especially) our mentors and spiritual
teachers. Bringing yoga into relationships has the power to change

us and how we are with others. Think about it—have you ever wished you could change someone else's behavior? And . . . how'd that work out for you? Probably not so good. But you *can* change your response to that behavior. In doing so, you can see beyond their actions to the person themselves. How can you do that? It begins by having a consistent personal practice, one that invites you to first cultivate a deeper understanding of what makes you . . . you. The more you get to know yourself, the easier it is to notice what's happening in your body—in real time—as you engage with another person or a group of people. You can listen for the meaning underneath the words and be able to respond appropriately—without immediately reacting or judging. You do that by accessing and checking in with the koshas—the five layers or sheaths that include and extend beyond our physical container. Whenever you come into a new situation and wonder if it's the right thing for you, do a little internal inventory based on the koshas, or energetic sheaths described in the Upanishads. Start by asking yourself what's going on with:

- **Your body (annamaya kosha, your physical body).** Do you feel at ease or fidgety? Do you have tension in your neck and shoulders or do your muscles feel pretty relaxed?
- **Your energy (pranamaya kosha, your breath and energy body).** Is your breath smooth or erratic? Or are you holding your breath?
- **Your state of mind (manomaya kosha, your thinking mind).** Do you feel calm and able to focus on the conversation or do you feel annoyed, agitated, or impatient? Or do you notice that your attention has drifted off somewhere else?
- **Your intuitive sense (vijnanamaya kosha, your wisdom body).** What does your inner wisdom or gut intuition tell you? Are you able to pause and listen before acting or responding?
- **Your deepest knowing (anandamaya kosha, your bliss body).** Do you feel a sense of joy and connection within yourself or with the person or group you're with? When

everything aligns, does your body feel at ease, your mind clear and focused, and your heart open and ready to receive?

NAVIGATING THE DIFFICULT MOMENTS

Dancing through the complex web of relationships in business, school, love, friendship, and parenting, we find yoga in not only those beautiful moments of connection but also moments where life isn't easy—where we're challenged or we feel our life is falling apart. Yoga often directs me to those times when I'm *not* mindful and invites me to notice how that affects my body, breath, mind, and heart. This is not new. Ever since the first yoga practitioners sat on their grass-woven seats to find peace, they too found challenges within their families, communities, and the world around them. The lives and stories of many of the early sramana forest practitioners (ascetics and wandering monks who rejected the authority of a very narrow version of Hinduism) demonstrate this, including Buddhists, Jains, and ajivikas. Siddhartha Gautama, the historical Buddha, of course, is the most prominent example for many of us.

Getting back on track requires that we return to the yamas, the ethical precepts we talked about at length in part 1. Although there are many different versions of the yamas, most traditions teach the yoga of kindness, non-harming, loving speech, deep listening, non-stealing, wise consumption, and nonattachment. Put into action, these codes are guides for how to behave with others. To care for and not hurt others: ahimsa. To speak kindly and tell the truth: satya. To not take or appropriate what belongs to others: asteya. To care for one's own energies: brahmacharya. To focus and let go of attachment: aparigraha.

Deepening our yogic path can sometimes cause us to fall prey to an enlarged ego, which can have a detrimental effect on our relationships. Especially if we start to think and act like we are somehow better—more accomplished, more centered, even more enlightened—than those around us. When that happens, I recommend rereading this quote by the spiritual teacher Baba Ram Dass: "If you're so enlightened, go spend a week with your family." I love this quote so much because so many of us have found ourselves humbled by experiences that remind us we still have far to grow. These moments give us an opportunity to pause and notice that our ego has "considerably overvalued its self-importance,"[1] as the spiritual teacher Rolf Sovik puts it, and regroup or perhaps find new ways to practice.

And speaking of family . . . the experience one of my esteemed colleagues shared with me is a perfect example of what I'm talking about. She told me that she's often challenged by the narrow definitions of what it means to be a woman in her very traditional family. She is a leader and visionary changing her field, but to her family, none of that means anything. They take great pains to remind her of her "place" as a daughter and a woman. So, when she's around them, she often finds her confidence shriveling. She tried all sorts of ways to convince her family that she is strong, capable, and successful. Until finally she decided to turn to her well-worn copy of the Bhagavad Gita. In the Gita she's reminded that, while it's imperative that we "engage fully in our actions" in what we're tasked to do, we must never equate our self-worth with how well we do those actions. When we overidentify with our "I-ness" (*ahamkara*), we separate rather than connect. In her desire for her family to see her worth as a successful leader—and be proud of her—she lost sight of the loving relationship she once had with them. We both agreed that sometimes it's in moments like these that we receive the greatest gifts—as long as we can stay open to learning. The challenging or difficult people in our lives, even as they are beloved, can be incredible teachers that invite us into our yogic practices.

⁘ A Mindful Relationship Practice

Our relationships can be deep teachers and give us opportunities to practice. Breathe and bring mindful awareness to how you can engage relationships we are born into and those we choose. Consider the following questions:

- What are the relationships that support your growth and spiritual evolution? Reflect on these. What do they have in

common? What sets them apart from other relationships that
may be more challenging?

• What are those more challenging relationships? Reflect on
how they can be teachers along your sadhaka path. What
yogic principles can you put into practice that will switch
them from challenging to workable?

• What qualities do you feel supported by in relationships?
Where are your growing edges?   ⠶

FINDING AND HONORING OUR TEACHERS ON THE PATH

Fully committing to a spiritual practice often means finding teachers, mentors, contemporaries, and wise elders along the path that
we can learn from, who can guide us and, when necessary, pick
us up when we fall, dust us off, and encourage us to keep going.
These days we have many ways of learning available to us. We can
learn from books, from teachers who teach online from thousands
of miles away, or from those who offer workshops, classes, or study
groups close to home.

For thousands of years, however, yoga could only be transmitted
orally from teacher to student. In fact, in the *guru-shishya* tradition,
one could not even practice without sitting at the foot of the teacher.
Many interpret this in a strict fashion in adherence to doctrine or
fundamental belief. There are still those today who say one should
not read or explore the texts without a learned teacher. I readily
admit that there are some wonderful and profound benefits to having a lineage and teacher. However, it's also important to note that
problems can and *do* arise with more high-demand or dominance-
oriented teaching styles, including exclusion, patriarchy, caste
oppression, and abuses of power. So it's important to note that you
don't have to adhere to a strict patriarchal relationship between
teacher and student or follow the call to a teacher in one particular
way. You don't have to buy into or go back to the behaviors and
constraints of a fundamentalist past. You get to choose the path
that is right for you. You may find classical training very valuable, or
you may gravitate to teachers who take a more liberal, poetic, and

metaphorical approach to the teachings. There are those who see guru—teacher—in nature, student, experiences, and in all. There are those who see guru within themselves.

The school of training I come from is a progressive Advaita Vedanta tradition with an emphasis on service and social engagement. It holds an inclusive, expansive, and liberal view. It is one where no one is deemed "wrong" for not having the proper pedigree. It is devoted to pre-Vedic inclusive yogic roots, process-based and growth-oriented in its perspective on lineage. Critical thinking and personal sovereignty are emphasized over adherence to tradition; caste and class do not matter, and no one is denied access to yoga or its teachings because of their social location. The Advaita Vedanta tradition sees all as developmentally appropriate and welcome to deepen in the practice. It invites all into yoga, regardless of time, place, space, material conditions, nationality, religion, race, class, gender, or any other factors; and it specifically practices yoga for personal and social liberation for all.

Think of your teachers—those you have sought out; those who have simply appeared when you were ready to receive them; those who have taught you yoga or invited you to dive deeper with yoga in your life; those you hope to study with and learn from. For some, this might be four or five people. For others, this may be thirty, or sixty—or too many to count.

We all have teachers. Call them to mind. What a joy to be able to learn from them. What gratitude pours out for those who have taught you. Your teachers are so precious. Take some time to thank them now in your heart and mind. Those teachers have teachers. Acknowledge the lineage and tradition. If your teachers are not from South Asia, it's likely that their teacher or their teacher's teacher was. If you go back far enough, you'll find yourself on the Indian subcontinent. For many generations teachers practiced in cities, in villages, under trees, and by rivers, seeking peace and freedom from suffering. They practiced finding truth, perhaps like you. And like you, some of these practitioners began to teach students. Some of those students became teachers themselves. The cycle of knowledge is passed on through time and space to come to you.

When I think about the relationships we make with our wise teachers and mentors, I imagine the profound ripple effect they have. I imagine a candle being lit, thousands of years ago, and passed down from teacher to student, until the light infusing that student spills over and into the world around them, touching friends, family, acquaintances, and even strangers they encounter during their day. Eventually this candlelight comes to you in an unbroken line of transmission of yogic wisdom. You are filled with the light of yogic knowledge. The more you learn, the more you practice, the more you embody yoga, the more your light glows. The light expands through every part of you, and from you it moves out into the world around you. You have become a transmitter of light through your every thought, word, action, and deed, and through the fights you defuse, the kind words you speak, the friends you help, the people you care for, and the students you teach. Your yoga is the yoga of relationships. It's not just something you *do*, it is something you *are*.

Hone Your Instincts and Beware False Gurus

It's not always easy to be discerning in relationships of the heart. Finding teachers, mentors, leaders, and even collaborators can be especially tricky. There are so many false gurus out there! It behooves us to choose our teachers wisely. Research a teacher or a practice that interests you—and talk with others you trust who have had experience with them. Transparency is key. No matter where that teacher comes from, no matter what lineage they carry or have been initiated into, if they abuse, cheat, lie, or engage in sexual misconduct, walk away. You do not have to see them as your teacher. In fact, they have disqualified themselves from being called teacher or guru; they are no longer worthy of your esteem as a teacher. You do not need to acknowledge those in your chosen lineage if they are abusive. You can still acknowledge your spiritual lineage, if you wish, by centering on those who came before them or simply refer to yoga as coming from the Indus Valley and Saraswati River Valley civilizations and people of India and South Asia.

Understanding the context in which abuse and harm happen does not excuse or justify the harm, which is always inexcusable, but bring awareness as to why certain things have occurred. In a colonial context, there has been so much suppression, harm, and trauma that those who existed under colonial rule often became tyrants even when "free" of that rule. This is part of how internalized oppression speaks like a snake in the heads of those who are oppressed. They internalize a sense of inferiority or shame and then replicate the harm enacted on them on others. Hurt people hurt people, as the adage goes. However, part of a sadhaka practice committed to ahimsa and other yogic values is to say "the harm stops here" and to work to transform harmful cycles into harmonious and healing ones.

Often the harm and abuse happen in cultures that create systems that perpetuate harm. As sadhakas, it's incumbent upon us to do what we can to change the culture in which those oppressive systems exist and replace them with ones that are more liberating. This is not at all suggesting that survivors are in any way responsible for the hurt inflicted upon them. Abuse, misuse of power, and false gurus should be addressed and stopped. Cultures of abuse and rape should never be part of yoga culture. Transparency, clear communication, community guidelines, and accountability go a long way toward creating more liberatory cultures.

Get a Perception Check

Just like in any kind of relationship, if something feels off or makes you uncomfortable, don't dismiss that feeling. Instead, listen to your intuition and check your perception. It's not that dissimilar to introducing your friends to a new love interest to get their read on what they observed or felt. I remember when I became interested in learning more about the Buddha's teachings. After all, the Buddha was a prototypical forest renunciate practicing yoga along with many other sannyasins seeking liberation and freedom from suffering. I had an opportunity to learn from Thich Nhat Hanh in person—and potentially immerse myself in the practice for a while— but I wanted to make sure I wasn't joining some kind of cult. I knew Hinduism from my heritage, but not much about Buddhism or his community of mindful practitioners. I wanted checks and balances on my own judgment. Thich Nhat Hanh was giving a talk nearby, so I asked my mom to come with me and to tell me what she thought. She agreed. I wanted her to get a feel for him—through his words and presence—to be better able to assess changes in me over the next several months.

I am lucky to have the kind of relationship with my mom where I can trust her to tell me straight, even if she doesn't agree with me. You don't have to rely on your mom as your check-and-balance measure, of course. It could be anyone whose judgment you feel you can trust. As it turned out, Thich Nhat Hanh put both of us at ease during his talk when he said, "No one should blindly follow a teacher, but actually, each one of us *is* the teacher!"

What this modeled for me was transparency and communication. For those of us who are in leadership roles in spirituality, yoga, mindfulness, meditation, or community space, we can continue to model this kind of practice. We can invite people to question us as teachers or mentors and to question the teachings themselves and our communities. We can host open Q&A sessions where we invite our students to ask us questions and share in exploration of the answers. We can invite people to join and explore. Let folks know they can bring other people with them—their therapist, friends, their mom . . . people they trust. We can invite prospective students to talk with current students. We can provide avenues for feedback and open space for discussion and critique. It is important to know you don't have to have all the answers. A great teacher or leader often doesn't! You can inquire with your community and point one another in the direction of more understanding. In cultivating such relationships, we deepen our relationship with one another—and with ourselves. We are in an ecosystem of care. We don't need to do any of this alone!

Find Someone Who Is Right for You

It's not always easy to find a teacher we resonate with—or a friend or romantic partner, for that matter; someone who is true, supportive, authentic, aligned, compassionate, and giving. When I first began dating, I remember thinking that there were no good examples of the kind of relationships I was interested in. I didn't see relationships of equality and shared power around me. So instead of looking to romantic relationships for my framework for how to be "in love," I looked to friendships. There I saw so many incredible examples of mutual support, interdependence, space, love, and uplift. I learned so much from my friends about how I wanted to relate romantically—as partners. In this same way, when looking for yoga teachers, spiritual teachers, or guides, it is important to consider what kinds of models we want to emulate.

No one wants to replicate abusive, top-down, power-driven, patriarchal, supremacist hierarchies; no one wants to sit at the feet of someone who tells them they're inferior and must only listen to what that teacher has to say. So what *do* we want? How can we know that a teacher is the right teacher for us; has our best interest at heart; and has the knowledge, qualities, and abilities that can support us as we learn? Here are a few guidelines I've used in finding a spiritual teacher. These are non-negotiables for me. You might also find them helpful in your search for collaborators, mentors, and others in leadership roles.

1. **Bring openness and inclusivity to your studentship.** Understand that you may have more than one teacher. In the traditional model, a lot of emphasis is put on finding one's singular teacher. However, historically, many yoga practitioners had multiple teachers and influences. This is true today. In fact, having multiple teachers can be quite healthy in a world that centers diversity. Be discerning. Take your time. Having multiple teachers can be wonderful when you allow their teachings to really water the seeds of your practice. Just be careful not to succumb to a kind of spiritual consumerism by seeing how many teachers you can accumulate to study with. Teachers are not acquisitions.

2. **Center the inquiry.** Look for teachers who don't insist they have (or that they are) the only truth. Instead, they invite their students into critical thinking about truth. Shankarji, one of my main yoga teachers in the Shankaracharya tradition, has been deeply influenced by J. Krishnamurti and

his emphasis on finding out for yourself what is true. He would present questions to us without offering any specific answers or solutions. We would debate, argue, puzzle, and mull over these questions for weeks. At first I expected Shankarji to eventually give us the "correct answer." But he never did! This is when I understood that for him, and the school of Advaita Vedanta he belongs to, the questioning and the inquiry are more important than any solution we seek. This is also a tradition I am grateful to pass on in my teachings with students. I remind my students that I'm sharing my experiences of how yoga has shown up in my life that gives rise to my own understanding. I invite them into their own inquiry to find self-sovereignty.

3. **Look for a sense of humor rather than "no ego."** Over the years of studying with masters in India and in the West, I have found that realized masters often have strong personalities. So I don't look for "no ego"—whatever that actually means! Instead, I look for teachers who have a sense of humor about their own personalities and foibles. For example, I can think of one master in the foothills of the Himalayas who used to giggle about her obsession with having a certain kind of herbal tea each morning before her sadhana. Being a tea lover myself, I was thrilled! I could really relate to her desire for tea in the morning. It was refreshing to hear her gently poke fun at herself for her attachment. Rather than pretending to be free of desires or above worldly concerns, she was perfectly human, just like me and the other students. And this made me trust her more when she taught us about detachment and wise action, because I knew she was working with and addressing this in her own practice.

4. **Someone who uplifts others.** I've noticed especially in the Western yoga space where we are practicing yoga or connecting yoga and social change that some people practice one-upping others or putting others down to distinguish themselves or make themselves look good. However, this ultimately only hurts the cause we are all working toward.

There are many ways to reach the same ends. We may differ in our modes and means, but the yogic way of honoring one another means we don't put down others. Instead, we recognize and acknowledge our differences rather than try to diminish them. This is a nuanced and important part of the practice. For example, you may see me critique *systems* that privilege some and exclude others, but I rarely critique people or schools because I feel it's more productive to work together on shared aims. I look for teachers and leaders who know who they are, know their values and work in integrity with those values, and recognize and uplift others doing similar work. I also look for those who refuse to talk badly about other teachers as this fosters distrust and division. (Caveat: Again, if you come across any teacher who causes harm through emotional or physical abuse, you have a responsibility not to shelter them. I believe transparency is key to changing cycles of abuse into cycles of healing and changing cultures for the better.)

5. **Someone I can trust.** I feel more fully myself when I'm in the presence of a teacher. I feel in my heart, gut, body, and brain who I can trust. I notice how it feels in my body around them. I notice when a teacher inspires inner confidence, calm, and peace; who radiates clarity, confidence, and compassion—and encourages the same qualities in their students.

6. **Look to the teacher within.** We may spend months or years looking far and wide to find the "right" teacher, only to realize that listening to tradition or learned teachers can only take us so far—that the truth, and perhaps even liberation itself, exists within. As Gautama Buddha, a prototypical yoga practitioner, is said to have reminded his followers, "Follow the truth of the Way. Reflect upon it. Make it your own. Live it. It will always sustain you."

⁜ Finding and Honoring Your Teacher Practice

- What do you look for in a spiritual teacher? Journal, reflect, discuss with a friend or colleague and express what you are looking for—and what you can't abide—in a teacher. Get specific! Talk it out, jot it down, or dance it.
- Once you think you've found a teacher—or even after you've been studying with someone for a while—it's good to check in with yourself. Close your eyes . . . feel what bubbles up for you when you recall the person or community you're considering. When you're around that person or in that community, notice what that feels like. Who are you in that space? Do you feel more like yourself? Is there a sense of spaciousness or contraction? Do you feel like a kinder, better version of yourself? Or do you feel judged or belittled in any way? Are there any red flags?
- Sometimes it can be helpful to pull out crayons and create a color story or mood board of the feelings in this experience. I find my body instinctively knows the way. By using my creativity to connect with my intuition, I am lead to experiences that support my growth and away from those that do not. ⁜

11

Moving into Conscious Leadership

Step 4

You are what your deep, driving desire is. As your desire is,
so is your will. As your will is, so is your deed. As your deed
is, so is your destiny.

—*KENA UPANISHAD*

HEEDING THE CALL to yoga, becoming a yoga steward, doesn't
mean you're suddenly an expert in all things yoga. It doesn't mean
you go out into the world and preach, hoping to convert the masses
to a particular way of life. It doesn't even mean you necessarily
become a yoga teacher. Rather, it means that your sadhana, your
spiritual practice, now informs everything you think, say, and do.
Trusting the deep connection you have with yoga allows you to
express it more fully in your daily life. The more you apply the teachings in your relationships, the more you can show up fully for the
benefit of *all* beings from a place of interconnection and love. How
do you do all that? How can you take your personal practice—the
investigation into "who you are"—and apply it to what you do? How
can you heed the call to selfless service (seva) that yoga sadhana
requires?

There are myriad ways to serve and make a difference in the
world. Don't get tripped up on having your activism—your way of
being a changemaker—look like someone else's path. All is welcome
when you choose to act in accordance with yogic principles, when

you discover your dharma. If you think you're not doing enough or will never be "that kind" of leader, let me tell you about Satish Kumar, an Indian-born Jain peace activist whose "small but beautiful" actions made a huge difference in the world.

When I met Satish Kumar, I could feel I was in the presence of someone living and leading their dharma. We sat in a circle in Navdanya, the Indian scholar and environmental activist Vandana Shiva's seed and soil preserving eco center at the foothills of the Himalayas. He shared his story of growing up Jain and described his mother and first spiritual teachers who taught him the ethos of doing no harm. I was rapt with attention as he spoke of the pilgrimage he took, determined to visit as many world leaders as he could, bringing tea and a message of peace. He left his home with no money and made it all the way around the world. By the time I met him, he was working in the United Kingdom, building small, transformative schools of social change in the heart of the British Empire. His edict was "small is beautiful," and he lived and breathed this message of social change—one relationship at a time.

The kind of leadership that Satishji embodies is based on undeniable integrity. All his actions revolve around his clear guiding principle of *small relationships build to great change over time.* From his early life to his current passions, everything is aligned in the embodiment of a leader who is truly living his teachings with such sweetness, humility, and joy.

We don't need to be Satish Kumar and do what he does to make a difference. We get to live into and lead from our own principles, influenced by our life experiences, our core competencies, and the skills we develop, as well as our unique nature. From such a place of self-awareness (svadhyaya), we begin to discover our true purpose, our dharma.

Dharma is another one of those words that has been co-opted by the Western world—along with *mindfulness* and *karma*—to such an extent that it's lost a lot of its original meaning and has plenty of questionable meaning layered onto it. I get it. It's really a hard word to define, so let's explore it together.

The Three Types of Dharma

First, dharma is not just one thing. In keeping with so many other concepts in yoga, it has multiple definitions. *Dharma's* root, *dhri*, translates as "that which upholds or maintains" or "that without which nothing can stand." I prefer to think of dharma as the universal or eternal law of nature. Why? Because such laws belong to the divine and cannot be manipulated by any religion or hierarchy of power. To attach any sense of sectarianism to the word *dharma* is to corrupt its meaning, writes S.N. Goenka, who was the foremost lay teacher of vipassana meditation. Dharma simply means *the cosmic order of things*. Goenka goes on to explain that dharma is what things *are* and what they *do*. For example, he says, the dharma of fire is to burn, and the dharma of ice is to be cold—forever and always. Fire is fire. Ice is ice. But that doesn't mean that dharma was ever meant to be a prescribed set of rules handed down by any person, religion, or institution. In its essence, dharma is a universal truth, or *sanatana dharma*—the eternal and unchanging nature of the universe.[1]

Samanya dharma relates to the moral and ethical codes that apply to everyone, which are outlined in the yamas and niyamas. These codes are not up for debate. The directives in them—such as non-harming, truthfulness, patience, generosity, justice, non-stealing, control of the senses, and dedication—give us a clear pathway for following our dharma.

Vishesha dharma is how you interpret the universal order as it applies to your life. It governs your duty to serve—and the way you serve—depending on your particular stage of life, and your interests and abilities.

Svadharma is how you choose to live your most conscious life. As the pioneer in integrative medicine Deepak Chopra writes, it's "the life you should be living."[2] It's your ideal life. Traditionally that ideal life meant living and serving in ways that aligned with your "predisposition at birth." The reasoning went like this: You could only be happy doing what you were meant to do, based on what you "came in with," so to speak. It really wasn't a matter of choice but rather a matter of not being fulfilled, not having "right livelihood," if you were to stray from your inherent nature. It wasn't until much later that the Brahminical patriarchy based it less on what you were born to do and more on what you were born *into*.

It can be difficult to sift through all the ways you may feel called to serve or to even think of anything you know how to do that would be of service to others! I've always found it helpful to return to my practice first—to get me fired up and ready to do something for the benefit of others. Sometimes just jumping onto my mat and doing asana—focusing on tapas (willpower), svadhyaya (self-discovery), and ishvara pranidhana (dedication)—provides the foundation I need to show up with fiery determination, steadfast commitment, and unconditional love.

The Pillars of Dharma

::

Just like in most yogic principles, there are many ways of characterizing the elements of dharma. Here are ten of the most common ones.

Patience	Sanctity
Self-Control	Truthfulness
Justice	Non-Stealing
Love and Dedication	Absence of Anger
Forgiveness	Spiritual Knowledge

:: Dharma Inquiry Practice

Think back on a time or two when you felt called to your purpose.

* Do you have a sense of your dharma, or are you still exploring it?

- What was happening in your life when you felt purposeful? What did that feel like?
- How did you answer the dharma call? Tell your story.
- What does the yogic way look like and feel like for you?
- Create an image of what it means for you to follow your dharma or be a vessel for yoga. Journal, paint, draw, or collage. Sculpt, dance, or play this vessel unique to your experience.

LEADING FROM YOUR ELEMENTAL NATURE

However we live our lives (our svadharma) and in whatever way we are meant to serve (our vishesha dharma), yoga meets us there and supports us along the path. Let's say you feel called to help stop the transmission of racism. Depending on who you are, where you're located, and what you feel your strengths and gifts are, this could mean getting loud, taking large and dramatic actions, and working on policy and culture shifts in organizations. Or it could mean working to change hearts and minds within your family, your partnerships, or in your local community. Some of us are comfortable going door to door with petitions to sign and discussions to have. Others would much rather be behind the scenes writing letters, making calls, volunteering at food banks, or marching on Washington, DC. A lot depends on your leadership style. If you're struggling to figure out what that is, you might find clues by getting to know your elemental nature. I'll explain.

Thousands of years ago, in Vedic times, yogis determined that everything in the world—all life—is made of five *tattvas*, or elements: *prithvi tattva* (earth), *aap tattva* (water), *agni tattva* (fire), *vayu tattva* (air), and *akash tattva* (space). Everything from our health and well-being to the way we live, practice, and lead is deeply impacted by which elements are most dominant within us. Over the years I've learned a lot about my leadership style by studying the Vedic model of the elements. Knowing our dominant elements can also help us know how to show up in the most loving and conscious way in our relationships. Take a read through the element descriptions here to see what resonates with you. I've even created a quiz on my website to help you identify your unique mind-body constitution and understand how you can best lead (YogaLeaderQuiz.com). It includes yoga tools and resources to support you, and practices tailored just for your leadership archetype, which will help you lead with more clarity, confidence, and power.

Earth

Some of us are earth element (prithvi tattva) yoga leaders. As an earth-based leader, you are known for channeling and harnessing the power of stability. You do best when you root into, live, and embody the heart of yoga practice. You communicate in ways that are calm, centered, nurturing, and wise. When you're in balance, you embody the qualities of groundedness, security, steadiness, connectivity. When you show up, you show up completely. Your growing edges might arise when you care too much or refuse to budge from a decision or opinion. Your imbalances show up as survival issues—when you are feeling ungrounded, stubborn, stagnant, or unable to let go or give up.

There are certainly some challenges to being an earthy leader. It can be a struggle to motivate yourself to get off the couch and get moving. You may need a vigorous practice to shake you out of your funk and get the energy flowing. But once you get started, you are solid, dependable, and grounded. Just like the planet Earth is brought alive by the rains, sun, and wind, you can turn to the other elements to enliven and invigorate your life. Connecting with folks who lead more with fire or air can be helpful to activate your grounded perspective.

Tune in to earth cycles and remember a grounded warrior is an effective and dependable leader. Always make sure you take some time to rest, ground, and get solid like a mountain before taking your next move. You are a planner—slow, thoughtful, and careful about how you work to make change. Love, trust, and follow your stability. It makes our world a better place.

Water

Some of us are wisdom changemakers filled with the water element (aap tattva). Your water-element power comes from going with the flow and being creative, inspired, and passionate about so many things. You do best when you are surrounded by water and able to share wishes and dreams with others. Supported by your yoga practice, you flow from one thing to another, moving with ease, integrating different streams of wisdom, learning, and practice into your life and work in the world. When you are in balance, you have a sense of abundance; you are full of creativity and confidence. Your growing edges might arise when limitations are imposed upon you, causing you to feel trapped, underestimated, or confined by too much structure.

Some say water-element leaders are flighty, flaky, or too "go with the flow." You can sometimes be a little hard to pin down. You may get overexcited by sensual pleasures and the finer things in life to the detriment of your ability to be practical or focused. When that happens, it's important to contain your flow. Just as a stream is defined by the banks that contain the river, you are supported by clarity, groundedness, boundaries, and guidelines. Connecting with those who are more earth-based can help you bring some solidity to your views and actions.

Your imbalances show up as flightiness, creative blocks, or a feeling of lack or scarcity. In those moments, a beautiful, flowing, fluid practice or visit to a body of water, stream, bath—or even drinking lots of water—can help shake you out of your funk! You can return to balance and your leadership qualities by tuning in to watery, flowy cycles and remembering a flowing water warrior is an effective leader. Take some time to recharge, nourish, and flow like a river before taking your next move. You can be quick to act when moved by new ideas and powerful moments in your work to make change. Follow your flow. Our world is better for it.

Fire

Some of us are the fire element (agni tattva) yoga leaders. Your power comes from your fiery inspiration, heat, light, and power.

Your words and actions ignite change. You do best when you are leading the charge and inspired for good in the world. You've got a vision, a plan, the motivation to make the world a better place, and the drive to get us there. You communicate in ways that are confident, leading, inspired, centered in your own power. You shine brightly.

When you are in balance, you are full of self-confidence, self-worth, and self-esteem, and your leadership is aligned in integrity and feelings of empowerment. Your growing edge might arise when you get so passionate that you lose nuance or perspective, you feel overpowered, you're focused without flexibility, or you're mired in perfectionism. Your imbalances show up as dominance, fear of being judged, lack of worth, insecurity, and a sense of failure.

Fire-element leaders often show up burning hot! Your vision and temper, as well as strong focus, can get you into trouble. These qualities can alienate you from other folks who don't share your intensity, passion, or views. Folks may feel you're taking over without listening or engaging others. Just as a fire is fed by air and contained by water, it's important for you to burn like a candle or campfire—not like a forest fire. You can turn to the wisdom of the other elements to support you; the perspectives of water- and earth-based leaders can be helpful in guiding your passion and tempering your immediacy.

In those moments where your fire is raging out of control, a calming and balancing practice can help you get back on track. Tune in to enlightened and bright cycles and remember a fiery warrior is an effective leader. Take some time to rest, ground, and get clear like a calm campfire or flickering candle before taking your next move. You make change by leading the charge to a better way, organizing protests and speaking up for justice or taking fiery and strong actions through letter writing or other means of sharing your strong opinions and feelings. Follow your fire. Our world needs it!

Air

Some of us are air element (vayu tattva) visionaries. As an inspiring air-element leader, your power comes from learning, strategizing, uplifting, studying, and sharing your insights. You do best when you are talking, visioning, and sharing ideas and dreams supported by the heart of yoga practice. You may be listening, expressing, organizing, and creating visionary movements. You have the vision to weave together many different streams of wisdom, learnings, and practice—yoga can support how you ideate and create in the world.

As for challenges to being an airy leader, you can be flighty, distracted, or kind of "on another planet." You can sometimes feel anxious, and your anxiety can cause you to talk too much, try to control people or situations, and take up a lot of space to feel safe. It's important to know when to get quiet and let the air flow into listening while others speak. It's not about biding your time until you get to share what's on your mind but rather listening deeply and allowing the quality of spaciousness to support your capacity to receive.

When you are in balance, you are full of trust, inspiration, love, joy, inner peace, kindness, and thoughtful care. Your growing edges arise when you feel overwhelmed or anxious, when there's too much structure and you're forced to focus on mundane things rather than visions and ideas, or when you are underestimated. Your imbalances show up as fear, lack of trust and feelings of being unlovable, unclear, confused, or clouded.

In those moments, a beautiful grounding practice can help you find stillness and calm. Staring at the moon or a lighted candle or having tea and conversation with a trusted friend can help shake you out of your funk and focus you as a force for good. Don't forget that you are supported by all the other elements, which can help you find your peace and clarity. Tune in to visionary, airy cycles and remember inspiring airy visionaries are effective leaders when calm, connected, inspired, and given space for their ideas to play! Take some time to listen, ideate, learn, nourish, and flow like a cloud in the sky before taking your next move. You're a dreamer with grand ideas for how to make change. Follow your visions. Our world needs them!

Space

Some of us are space-element (akash tattva) leaders. As such, your power comes from being in tune with energy, spiritual nourishment, and forces beyond what we can see. You do best when you live and embody the spiritual heart of yoga practice. You are at your clearest when you are listening to the true, clear, interconnected voice within. You are calm, spiritually centered, solid, nurturing, and wise. Your qualities in balance are connection to spirit, the present moment, service, spirituality, and pure bliss!

Your growing edge may arise when you feel completely disconnected, purposeless, and nihilistic. When that happens, it's hard to be in your power and truth. Your leadership can feel off the mark, too idealistic, or just not in alignment with others. Connection with the perspectives of the other elements can bring you back to earth.

When you're out of balance, you can feel like your life has no meaning and you've lost your sense of connection to the divine. In those moments, a strong, dedicated meditation or gentle inversion-filled Hatha Yoga practice can help bring you back to your spiritual center. Just as space is defined by the objects that fill it, you find your meaning and purpose in the challenges that arise in life. Often it's right in the heart of our disenchantment that our deepest truths and insights are born. Take some time to meditate, tune in, trust your intuition, and get clear and spacious before taking your next move. You might be tuned in to spiritual insights that help our world and naturally evolve us to make change for the better. Follow your spirit. Our world is so much better for it!

Remember to visit YogaLeaderQuiz.com to help you understand how you lead best. You'll get personalized yoga tools and resources for your unique leadership style and practices for your leadership archetype to help you lead with more ease, clarity, and confidence.

Sadhakas Speak: Sadhaka Shyam Ranganathan

::

My sadhana is philosophy. It is a disciplinary practice that forces one to own one's own choices (svadhyaya) while challenging oneself to understand beyond past choices (tapas) while learning to get along with others in a world of quirky individuals.

—Shyam Ranganathan, MA, PhD

12

Self-Care as We Serve

Step 5

Caring for myself is not self-indulgence, it is self-
preservation, and that is an act of political warfare.
—AUDRE LORDE, *A BURST OF LIGHT*

BEFORE WE EXPLORE all the ways yoga can support our work in
the world, let's examine what can get in the way of doing that work
in the first place. Yoga doesn't make us immune to challenges in the
world. Even the most committed practitioner can get overwhelmed
and become emotionally and physically exhausted to the point of
burnout. I know that *burnout* is one of those words that gets thrown
around a lot. But what is it really and how does it impact our ability
to show up fully as ourselves in service to the causes we believe in
so fervently?

Psychology Today defines burnout as "a state of emotional, mental, and often physical exhaustion brought on by prolonged or
repeated stress."[1] Though it's most often caused by problems at work,
it can also appear in other areas of life, such as parenting, caretak-
ing, or romantic relationships. We've all experienced times of stress:
when we have difficult conversations with our partner, our kids, or
a teammate; when we're working for social justice causes and feel
like we're not getting anywhere; when we are struggling to meet
an impossible deadline. Stress can make us feel frantic, anxious, or
overwhelmed. Burnout is different. Although it can certainly be the
result of unrelenting stress, burnout is a state of being "all dried up."

As stress worsens into burnout, it's common to lose focus, interest, and motivation for work, relationships, and projects. It's pretty terrible. It can drain your energy and can make you feel hopeless, helpless, cynical, and lost, which are all understandable feelings in the world we live in. However, with the tools of yoga, we can always take positive personal steps toward well-being. Practicing svadhyaya, in particular, can help us become aware of early warning signs—those "beige" flags—of burnout before they become red flags, an SOS emergency call. Our bodies, minds, and spirits give us many subtle and not-so-subtle signs we can heed if we truly listen.

How Do You Know You're Moving toward Burnout?

People experience burnout in different ways, so know that the following flags are just my suggestions for what to pay attention to. And keep in mind that any yoga wellness or health advice presented here is not meant to replace the advice of your personal physician or other health-care professional, so always seek competent medical care.

Beige/Red Flags—Physiological Signs
- Your body, shoulders, neck, lower back, chest, or feet start to hurt all the time.
- Your life energy feels blocked.
- You seem to come down with a cold or flu more often.
- You are tired, with low energy or completely exhausted.
- You are not breathing deeply.
- You are not getting enough good nourishment or sleep.

Beige/Red Flags—Mental and Emotional Signs
- Your feelings seem overwhelming or, conversely, you feel flatlined.
- Your mind and heart are full of tension, stress, or irritation.
- You're unclear about—or beginning to doubt—your purpose.

- You feel out of sync with intuition and higher purpose.
- You feel like you are in a pressure cooker.
- You get down or easily upset.
- You feel unsupported and unheard.
- You often feel frustrated and overwhelmed.

What Does Healthy Balance Feel Like?

Knowing or remembering how it feels to be in balance can help you notice when you are moving more toward imbalance. These green flags can be helpful checkpoints to pay attention to.

Green Flags—Physiological Signs
- Your body feels healthy and strong for you.
- You can listen for and respond to your body's cues.
- There's tension but it doesn't feel stuck—it's moving.
- Your creativity feels alive, open, and flowing.
- You feel energized and you're eating well for you.
- Your breathing is full and deep.
- You stand fully open and tall.

Green Flags—Mental and Emotional Signs
- You feel calm and centered, happy, and joyful.
- You pay attention and respond to how you're feeling.
- You experience peace, flow, and grace.
- You are in sync with your intuition and higher purpose.
- You are secure in your worthiness.
- You feel confident and in flow.

How best to move from red to beige and ultimately to green? By prioritizing self-care. I know, I know—for many of us, self-care has become somewhat of a joke. It's portrayed as self-serving and even selfish. For many of us, self-care has become synonymous with a capitalist fixation on goodies and perks. But taking care of yourself is *not* selfish. You need to care for yourself so that you can be there to sustain your energy, therefore you can show up at your fullest for your community and the causes that need you. Now that I've made my case, let's connect the two.

SELF-CARE IS VITAL FOR SOCIAL JUSTICE

Self-care, care for others, and social change are interconnected. There has been a legacy of leadership around the interconnectedness of self-care and social justice particularly led by queer Black women, beginning with Audre Lorde in the early 1980s. In a speech at Harvard University in 1982, Audre Lorde made the radical, paradigm-shifting statement that "there is no such thing as a single-issue struggle because we do not live single-issue lives."[2] Six years later, soon after she was diagnosed with cancer for the second time, Audre Lorde wrote perhaps one of her most quoted lines: "Caring for myself is not self-indulgence, it is self-preservation, and that is an act of political warfare."[3]

Within systems that are not built for our well-being, caring for ourselves is an incredibly radical act and a powerful part of social justice. Watered-down self-care that is more about feeding a capitalist idea of what we need to buy in order to feel good distorts the true meaning of self-care. Authentic self-care, on the other hand, nourishes us and supports our work in the world.

Not that long ago, a yoga colleague was experiencing a lot of anxiety at the constant pressure to produce, perform, connect, serve others, and . . . be perfect. "It's just not possible, is it?" she asked me one afternoon as we hiked. "It's not," I replied. I told her that perfection is an illusion and a tool of systems of oppression to make us feel like we are wrong, flawed, not doing enough. I went on to say that these systems are really set up so we can never do all the things required or demanded of us in the first place—and still be fully human. We talked about all the ways yoga practice could support her. As we checked in from time to time, she reported that prioritizing pranayama practices like *sama vritti* (equal breathing), as well as a slow, earth-based, gentle vinyasa helped her shift her nervous system away from a breakdown state toward a more harmonious one.

Recommitting to her meditation practice allowed her to focus her attention and not succumb to the cultural pressure of multitasking. We both agreed that paradoxically, the more present and fulfilled we were, the more we could actually accomplish.

It's almost a cliché to say that we can't possibly take care of others without first taking care of ourselves. But it's true. Why? Because when we take the time to care for ourselves—to deeply rest our body and our mind—we are better able to show up grounded, with a clear mind and more patience. When we feel centered within ourselves, we can more readily be there for others—without internal distractions. When we find inner peace, we can participate in creating outer peace.

In her book *Self Care Matters: A Revolutionary's Approach*, the strategic self-care consultant Anana Johari Harris Parris describes self-care as "any act that addresses needs in regular and critical areas of your life." She breaks it down into six categories: spiritual/emotional, economic (money, energy, time), artistic, physical, educational, and social. In combining spiritual and emotional care, Harris Parris makes a case for how connected our emotions and sense of meaning are. We can care for ourselves spiritually by nourishing our personal growth. Emotionally, we can care for ourselves, she explains, "by being aware of our emotions, experiencing what comes up for us without judgment, and being more tender, loving, and patient with ourselves." She goes on to say that we care for ourselves economically by making sure we have enough time, energy, and money to support our needs; artistically, by giving our creative expression space to play; physically, by giving our body what it needs in terms of rest, sustenance, movement, and pleasure; educationally, by making a commitment to learning and expansion. And, finally, we care for ourselves socially by interacting in ways that nourish us and support our own and on another's growth in the other five areas of self-care. Each of these self-care commitments is important so we can continue to nourish ourselves while we do the work we are here to do in the world. As Harris Parris shows us, self-care is not simplistic but rather complex and filters outward in a powerful way.[4]

Think of self-care as an act of metta, maitri, and karuna—love, care, and compassion—a love letter to yourself and in service to others. It is a way of centering a physical practice that allows you to move, stretch, and discover places in your body that need to release tension; a breath practice that helps harmonize your nervous system; a way to clear your mind, solve problems, and respond from the *whole* of you to the circumstances around you. It can also help you home in on your purpose, your svadharma, and come into a clearer alignment with your values and truths. Once established in your purpose, self-care becomes a way of refilling the coffers of the heart and mind so that others may benefit as well.

Self-care is a lever in a much bigger system. We aren't suggesting that anyone stop with just self-care—that's self-indulgence. Self-care is interwoven with how we nurture our relationships and engage in making the world a better place.

A Few Simple Self-Care Practices

What can you do to move your self-care dial from red to green? Here are a few simple things I've found that I can easily call upon when I need to recalibrate—or better yet, fold into my day before stress overtakes me. First, when things get really difficult, I cancel my appointments, lie down, and put my legs up the wall or go to sleep. The call is to change your awareness toward recharging yourself— for example, by taking a shower or a little nap. Whatever helps you shift into a new state of energy and awareness. Even if you only have five minutes between obligations, lie down on the earth for a gentle recharge. If you have more time, take a brisk afternoon walk or do an afternoon yoga nidra practice for twenty to thirty minutes, which allows you to move into deeper states of consciousness. Start your morning (or finish your day) with some pranayama or journaling. Or try abhyanga oil massage, an Ayurvedic practice where you gently and caringly massage a natural oil, such as coconut or sesame oil, into your skin. Chanting mantras or doing a short mudra or asana practice for a few minutes can also help care for oneself. It doesn't have to be fancy! Try on a few of these practices and see how you feel.

Self-Care through Connection and Play

There's a common belief among trauma experts that we suffer in isolation and we heal in community. It stands to reason, then, that a vital part of our self-care routine should include connecting with others—talking, laughing, singing, playing, sharing our lives. I think of this lightness of being as tending to the heart and stoking the spiritual fire of our sadhana. Making an effort to be close to people and things that nurture our spiritual growth is important. As the South African theologian and archbishop emeritus Desmond Tutu once said, "I can be human only in relationships. Our greatest good is communal harmony." Being present with colleagues, mentors, or friends who embody elements of the practice is powerful. Whenever I've met, or had the privilege of connecting with, students and colleagues who embody yoga—or studying with spiritual teachers, such as Shankarji, Kabirji, my dharma teachers; the Dalai Lama; or Thich Nhat Hanh—I notice they have a tremendous sense of humor and play, what yogic texts call *lila*.

Lila in Sanskrit is richer and deeper in meaning than "play" or "sport." It means taking delight in the present moment as well as the eternal and the unending play of God or the divine. It can also mean divine love.

In the play of the universe that is constantly involved in creation, destruction, and re-creation, there is a lightness and humor that can arise within deep yoga practice.

Over years of practice, I learned to notice this lila, or play, within myself. Rather than acting in ways that were anxious or uptight, like I did when I was younger, more and more I felt like someone who could go with the flow, tap into her presence and power, speak up or listen, and smile at the joys and even the sorrows of life.

I was so in love with the practice I went on retreat after retreat, and this allowed my practice to mature and deepen. I remember some other young folks new to the practice of yoga and meditation. They were on their first retreat and feeling so giddy and hyped up. One of our teachers was watching them one morning, during the first month of their stay at the ashram, and said, "Your joy right now is still on the surface. It will deepen. You don't have to try so hard or hold on to it so much."

I watched their faces fall a bit. After all, they *did* feel joyful and elated. At the same time, what our teacher said was certainly true. While joy can and does bubble up and it feels amazing, it's so much more than that. Be patient and keep practicing—the more you commit to studying and embodying the eight limbs over time, the more lila can deepen into a wise, embodied companion that lives in your soul, bones, and behind the crinkles around your eyes and smiling mouth.

Your connection to yoga, your sadhaka journey, is unique to you. But inviting in a sense of playfulness and fun, of emanating respect while also not taking your practice or yourself too seriously, can bring a soft, connected way of being. You might find that connection to practice through a spiritual friend or a beloved community. You might find your doorway is grief or anger or joy or gladness. There will be those who really nurture your spiritual growth and path. Recognize and nourish those relationships. For example, I have a daily practice, spiritual practice buddies I chat with weekly, and a sangha practice space I gather in each week to explore yogic values. I also take myself on a retreat at least once a year—even if it is a solo retreat that I curate for myself over a weekend. All of these practices stoke and tend my spiritual fire.

⁚⁚ CONNECTION AND PLAY INQUIRY PRACTICE

- What are some connection practices that can support your spiritual growth?
- Where do you notice lila the most in your life? The least? Where do you think you can call in more joy and play into your life?
- Think of a way you can express the sense of lila that yoga arouses in you. Perhaps through dance, writing, singing, or spending time in nature.

SADHAKAS SPEAK: AARTI INAMDAR

⁘

At the moment, my sadhana includes personal practice along with support for my life as a householder. I first noticed the shift when I was pregnant. I found myself practicing with additional intentions that included the well-being of my growing baby. I could no longer practice just for me. Much like motherhood was a rebirth for me, the same rebirth happened with my sadhana, which had shifted to include the health and well-being of my family. Now as a householder yogi with two beautiful children, I still practice with my personal ultimate goals in mind, along with the intention to support the health and well-being for me and my family. As I fulfill my responsibilities as a parent, partner, daughter, sibling, businessperson, and yoga teacher, I lean on my sadhana to support me fully. Sadhana shifts over time, I've learned to adapt to and love those changes.

—Aarti Inamdar, MSc, BMC

⁘ SELF-CARE REFLECTIONS

- What is one action you can take right now to practice care for your own body?
- Thinking about your personal practice, what do you turn to (readings, mantras, music) that helps ground and support you?
- Whom do you turn to when you need a listening ear? And how can you be that for others in your community?
- How does caring for yourself support and contribute to your service in the world?   ⁘

∷ Is It Self-Care or Selfish?

Here's a practice I've done in class to examine the difference between selfish acts and acts of self-*care*. You'll need four blank pages in your journal: label the first one "Selfish," the second one "Self-Care," the third one "Self-Indulgence," and the fourth one "Service." To get started, spend some time and list everything you can think of that connects you to each category. Everything. Don't think too hard; just write. Here are some sample questions to begin!

- **Selfish.** What does selfish mean to you? List some of the ways you're selfish. What does "selfish" feel like in your body?
- **Self-Indulgence.** What does being self-indulgent mean to you? List some of the ways you indulge yourself—some of your secret pleasures. What does it feel like after it's over?
- **Self-Care.** What does self-care mean to you? List some of the ways you practice self-care. When you practice self-care, what does that feel like?
- **Selfless Service.** What does truly serving others—with no expectation of reward—mean to you? List some of the ways you serve (or wish to serve)—in the smallest of ways and in the grandest. What does selfless service feel like? How does it differ from self-indulgence?

After diving into these questions, reflect on what you included, perhaps what you left out, and what came up for you. Which categories were easy to populate? Which ones were a struggle? I noticed when I did this exercise that I didn't want to focus my time or energy on the things I put in the "Self-Indulgence" column. But much of what I listed in the "Selfish" column was actually essential to self-care! Like taking time for myself; space to be in water or take a bath. And I had the aha realization that if I didn't do those things, I wouldn't be nourished enough to do the things that live in the "Service column." What were your *ahas*?   ∷

SADHAKAS SPEAK: NIKKI MYERS

⁙

My life's work revolves around healing my own and supporting others to heal various forms of addiction. This encompasses not only substance abuse or behavioral compulsions but also our addiction to specific ways of perceiving reality. Lasting recovery from addiction demands an exploration into the intricate layers of *samskaras*, our ingrained habits and patterns, and *vasanas*, our subconscious tendencies.

I use regular practice to refine my ability to delve into these depths. Sadhana plays a pivotal role in broadening my capacity to embrace complexities and seeming contradictions.

In a way, it parallels vital routine acts like brushing my teeth or combing my hair. However, more than a routine, sadhana weaves a connection between my inner being and external reality.

And much like life itself, my sadhana changes. Sometimes it varies from day to day or season to season. Regardless of its form, whether a five-minute pause (what I call a yoga snack) or an hours-long practice, my sadhana encompasses some blend of asana, pranayama, and meditation.

Sadhana then becomes this sacred bridge, guiding me with grace and mindfulness through life's complexities. It's a profound journey that helps me navigate life with resilience and a more peaceful flow of inner awareness.

—Nikki Myers, founder Y12SR; IAYT yoga therapist

13

Collaborating with Allies on the Path

Step 6

Sa tu dirgha kala nairantarya satkara adara asevita drdha bhumih
To achieve a strong foundation in our practice, we must practice over a long time, without interruption, believing in it and looking forward to it, with an attitude of service.

—YOGA SUTRAS

IN ALL THE YEARS I've been doing this work, I don't think I've ever heard anyone say that living their yoga as spiritual practice was easy. Because it's often not! Sometimes it just feels like too much—too hard to sustain, too confusing, even too lonely. Indeed, the pull to give up begins almost immediately after we step over that threshold and say yes to being an agent of spiritual possibility, a true sadhaka. *What was I thinking? I'm too busy. I don't know enough. I don't even know where to start.* Such moments (days, weeks, years) of resistance can be hard to . . . well, resist. If this has been your experience, you're in good company. And like everything in life, remember, it's not permanent.

I've found that the antidote to all these "too muches" is connecting with others; calling in your allies and being an ally as well. I bet, if you really think about it, you'll find there are many who are with you on your journey. Allies are powerful because they remind us that we are not alone.

What exactly is an ally? In its very basic form, an ally is that friend, mentor, or teacher who can shore you up when you're down, guide you home when you're lost or confused, and offer advice when you're struggling or stuck. You do this for others too. We learn how to act as an ally by bringing our values into alignment with our actions—in other words, living the yogic precepts (the yamas and niyamas). An ally can be someone (or something) who supports your personal, emotional, intellectual, and spiritual growth; a community of presence and practice that will, if you wish, hold you accountable. We all need allies, and our yoga practice guides us to receive the support and—equally important—to offer such support to others.

I like to think of *ally* as a verb as well, because it's something we *do* as much as it is something we *are*. We ally ourselves with others, with causes, with justice. It's an intentional choice that's not focused on our identity but rather on our actions. Allying ourselves with others allows us to act in a way that serves the greater good without getting our ego wrapped up in the outcome. To be an ally is to be willing to leverage one's privilege to address structures and systems where others are marginalized—and to stand up for the individuals who are being marginalized or harmed. It is a willingness to reach across differences to support members of a community other than one's own and, at times, to achieve a mutual goal. For example, a teacher who speaks up on behalf of a student who repeatedly gets detention for being late to school. Using their authority, the teacher can intercede, letting the powers that be know that the student works before school, thereby helping to ensure that the student receives understanding instead of punishment. Straight parents, teachers, friends, and other members of the community can be allies for the LGBTQ+ community, by sharing their pronouns and speaking up to interrupt homophobia and heteronormativity. There are many ways to be an ally. Finding and creating allies is one way to live our yoga.

Finding Allies

Part of your practice is remembering how connected you already are. We are all connected through the earth that we are sitting, standing, and walking upon. We are connected through the moon and stars above our heads. We are connected through touching the truth and our love of the practice. We are connected through shared experiences, through our humanity. This connection has always been there; it's just that sometimes we forget. You may find glimpses of it in a conversation with a friend, a family member, a teacher. Even some random person you see on the street who says something in passing that makes you smile can somehow make the world come back into focus. You may find it in nature, in a moment of complete connection with all that is. Remember, too, that your family (blood-related or chosen) and your ancestors can be powerful allies when you call them in.

Allies come in many forms; they don't always have to be people. Sometimes a book, a poem, a passage from a sacred text, or a piece of music can speak to you in a way that helps you remember who you are. Intangible things can also be allies. Energies can be allies. That sweet taste of the pause you savor when you look up and see a ray of sunlight breaking through the fog on a challenging day. Those moments in which you are able to sit in silence, with your journal by your side, and sip from the warm cup of tea. The place you choose to roll out your mat—under the stars, on the sand near the ocean, or in your messy living room; anything, no matter where you are, that allows you to touch into a segment of your deep inner peace. An ally can be anything that offers you space and permission to pause or go deeper into your practice of living your yoga, your truth.

We can take on grand gestures and go on retreats or pilgrimages. These are large and public intercessions that interrupt life as usual and invite complete shifts and transformations. We can quietly and privately experience the allyship of a guided meditation or a yoga nidra session. Even sadness, pain, loss, and grief can be gentle guides into deeper practice.

As you reflect on these connections, think about how they show up in your life. Notice them. Celebrate them! Reflect on where you'd like to call them in more. Maybe even notice your reluctance to reach out to your allies or to offer yourself up as an ally to others. Yoga itself is *yuj*, "union." All of our experiences, allies, and communities we are part of can show us the way back to union within ourselves, with one another, and with the world around us.

It's not always easy to receive the gifts an ally can bring, especially in European cultures that pride themselves on being independent, go-it-alone types. Sometimes, as I discovered in India, they show up anyway, in the most unlikely ways. Four at a time!

I was in Bodhgaya, Bihar, not far from the School of Minds my father had attended as a teenager. As a young teacher now myself, I had been asked to come to a local village school and share some teaching methodologies with the faculty.

While working there, practicing austerities was part of the job description. I stayed in a simple village complex where three other workers at the school lived. One was a Buddhist monk. Another was a Hindu sannyasin (renunciate). The third was a young teacher from Sandiya, a small village north of Bodhgaya.

We came together to plan our training for the faculty and at mealtimes. The conversations we had over those meals! I learned about everything from freedom fighting to Vedic astrology from my three teachers. Their wisdom—whether it was village wisdom or Buddhist or Hindu scripture and practice—was incredibly supportive to a simple life full of spiritual practice.

I learned from a fourth teacher as well: Bodhgaya itself. Pilgrims come from all over the world to visit the Mahabodhi complex, a large brick enclave surrounding the large Bodhi Tree that lives there, a descendant of the one that the Buddha sat under and attained enlightenment, thousands of years ago. Bodhgaya was a teacher to me in many ways. Witnessing the depth of devotion that all the spiritual seekers—Hindu, Buddhist, Muslim—brought to their places of worship. At 5:00 a.m. the call to prayer was heard along with chants to Shiva and the Lotus Sutra. Sacred sounds of devotion continued throughout the day and into the night. The interfaith care and cooperation I experienced from villagers there showed a possibility of yoga in action I hadn't experienced before.

During my time there, I managed to get a parasite. It didn't seem to bother me too much. I was tired, but the antibiotics I took after more natural approaches had failed seemed to do the trick. I figured

I was fine, and anyway, I was fiercely independent and didn't think what I was experiencing was worth sharing.

On a particularly hot day, the monk, the sannyasin, and I decided to take a walk from the temple to Dungeshwari (about five miles from the Bodhi Tree). We headed out early to avoid the heat. The path was long and winding, through villages and across the stream near where the Buddha felt faint from malnourishment after years of austerities; where Sujata, a village girl, brought him water and *kheer*, a sweet rice like my father used to make when I was ill or needed comfort. Her actions revived the Buddha; he was able to recover and realize the Middle Way.

As we reached the dark caves, I marveled at a culture where conversations about liberation and practices to support it were so prevalent. I felt a bit faint as we walked the six or so miles back to Bodhgaya. By the time we got home, the temperature had soared to 110 degrees, and I was dizzy, sick, and unable to function.

Marveling at how my own walking path had in some small way mirrored that of the Buddha's, I collapsed onto my bed to rest. Rest was not to be, however. I was so feverish I began talking nonsense, and the local village teacher who stayed with us ran to get the monk and sannyasin to see if they could help. I was burning hot and yet I could not stop shivering.

I could hear one of the clinicians say something like, "I think her organs are shutting down." But in my fevered state I couldn't respond. All I could hear was Hindu slokas and Buddhist mantras being chanted above me. It was a strange and distressing night. As dawn broke, so did my fever and I was able to truly rest. My dear friend and colleague stayed with me, putting cool rags on my brow and offering words of encouragement through the morning until I was cooler. She was a true spiritual friend, a *kalyanamitra*. Through her actions and those of my other allies, I came to realize my own middle way of interdependence rather than fierce independence. From my experience in Bodhgaya of near death and great physical distress, I gained an embodied knowledge of surrender and true allyship and support.

Being an Ally

Allyship goes in all directions. Not only will you be enriched by having allies but being an ally for others can lead you into seva (selfless service), where you may find that there's no longer any difference between giving and receiving. Perhaps there's an ecosystem, an animal, or a cause you're passionate about—and you want to offer your service. Remember the golden rules of allyship: be humble, practice deep listening, and present your truth (satya) laced with love (ahimsa) so you don't become a savior rather than an ally.

In social justice work we make a distinction between being an ally and being an accomplice. To be clear, both are important. The most common way to explain the difference is that an ally is someone who stands with—or often intercedes on the behalf of—a marginalized person or community. In other words, an ally uses their privilege for good rather than to harm. An accomplice will work *with* an individual or group to dismantle the systems or structures that created the imbalance in the first place. According to the educator, organizational leader, and fundraising/communications strategist Jonathan Osler, who wrote the guide "Opportunities for White People in the Fight for Racial Justice," an accomplice's actions "are informed by, directed and often coordinated with leaders who are Black, Brown, First Nations/Indigenous Peoples, and/or People of Color."[1] For example, white people can be true allies for BIPOC by analyzing and addressing lack of diversity in the workplace, schools, or the wellness industry. They can also be accomplices by taking action to lobby organizations, politicians, and corporations to propel them to change the system.

In the yogic context, an ally might educate themselves on the issues of cultural appropriation and the need to honor yoga's roots. An accomplice would, once they have educated themselves, act to dismantle the practice by working alongside the teachers who are leading the way in these conversations. Consider the student who was deemed delinquent for repeatedly getting to school late. Their teacher showed up as an ally, interceding on the student's behalf to protest the punishment and have it overturned. An accomplice could take that one step further by working to dismantle the rule that made the student's detention mandatory in the first place. Once again, both are important and necessary.

I first heard the language of allyship in the intentional spiritual activist community I built in Los Angeles in 2001–2015. We put the work of being allies into practice working across differences to uplift one another. For example, as allies we supported each other across different identities. Some of our white members learned a lot about systemic racism. We were all committed to educating ourselves and others. However, we soon realized that allyship was not enough; we needed to develop tools and practices for being accomplices. For example, as allies we were learning all we could about the school-to-prison pipeline. For the folks who were living it, they needed us to step up as accomplices and raise bail funds and money for legal fees, show up at court dates, and write letters to support our members of color who were dealing with the criminal justice system. From our different positionalities we all worked to overturn laws that were propping up the school-to-prison pipeline. This is a continued and evolving exploration—allyship and accompliceship are continued actions and not a final destination!

WHEN SELF-DOUBT GETS IN THE WAY

The practice of yoga teaches us how to be allies to others as well as how to look for and find allies for ourselves. The allies I find along the path are part of what makes the work I do easier and more enjoyable, and they can bring solace in times of despair and challenge. Yet committing to allyship or accompliceship can be nerve-racking, especially if you're a bit out of your comfort zone. The question I get often from folks stepping into the work is, "How can I do this work without it getting overwhelming or harming myself?" And, of course, the big one: "How can I do this work without messing up?"

Let's get the latter question taken care of right away. You will mess up. We all do. Chances are good that most of us will at times act in ways that aren't in alignment with our values and that don't support the folks we stand with. If that happens, what can you do? Acknowledge, apologize, and learn from your mistakes. The key to being a conscious ally or accomplice is being self-aware. We must look within, recognize when we're out of alignment, and commit to doing the work to come back into integrity. It also can be possible to take on a little bit of discomfort, to feel out of your element, in order to alleviate other people's pain. This is part of the work of being an ally and accomplice. The key is to remember to take care of yourself along the road to creating change.

You may have feelings or thoughts along the way that you're not proud of. That's normal too. When we live inside of (and benefit from) systems that perpetuate discrimination and harm, it would be impossible not to. It's critical that you notice, name, and own them—without shame or blame, neither of which is helpful. Think of these uncomfortable thoughts and feelings as allies on your sadhaka path—inviting you to stop, listen, and recalibrate. Your commitment to ahimsa, satya, and ishvara pranidhana—love, truth, and devotion—begins with yourself. Despite the countless times you'll "mess up," you are inherently divine.

Mindful Collaborations

An important way to support others as an ally—and be supported by allies yourself—is to collaborate. By being part of a group dedicated to a common cause, working together and sharing the load, you can increase the possibility of effecting change and perhaps decrease the possibility of burnout. I used to think that all it took was for collaborators to be on the same page, feel that sense of urgency and dedication to a cause, and things would work smoothly. Of course, it's never that easy. As with most things, I've seen and been a part of some incredible collaborations and some really challenging ones. The challenging ones can often be good teachers; they help us learn what *not* to do. Here's a case in point.

Two yoga teachers came together to create a special yoga workshop. They both agreed on the subject matter but hadn't really taken the time to discuss their assumptions or expectations. In their excitement, they jumped right into planning and making things happen. It didn't go so well. One person was tasked with doing all the detailed work—creating fliers, writing the copy, posting on social media, sending out email reminders, and even processing payments. The other person didn't do any of the work but would often complain about the work that their partner did.

The workshop itself was a great success. They had about twenty participants. However, the teacher who hadn't done any of the prep work took over, leading the workshop and relegating the other teacher to an "assistant" role. From start to finish this collaboration was rocky and imbalanced. I heard about it from the hardworking partner, who eventually let their cofacilitator know their concerns. They also admitted they had learned a lot from the experience, including how important it is to enter into a collaboration with care, after thinking a lot about what you want in a partner—and to be clear about who does what, when, and how much. The duo decided to keep the split fifty-fifty but to never collaborate again.

On the flip side, I can personally attest that collaborations can be absolutely magic. A great collaboration is always far more than the sum of its parts. This year I had the privilege of collaborating with some old colleagues as well as new friends to create a fundraiser for a powerful cause. We came together in a small Palestinian and Black-owned arts and movement space in South Los Angeles and created a space founded in yogic ethics and practices. A colleague brought in art as a tool of resistance, protest, and changing the narrative. Two other colleagues led a circle for mindful sharing. The whole experience was incredible, and I loved learning from my cofacilitators for a good cause. When two or more people come together in a complementary way, they round out an experience and bring life and magic to it. I've seen this work so well when people collaborate with folks who have skills and abilities they don't. For example, when a person who is vision- and idea-driven collaborates with someone who is grounded, practical, and action-oriented—that's when magic happens. This doesn't mean everything always happens smoothly. It rarely does. In fact, having good communication, a backup plan, and a process for what to do when a team hits conflict is key to successful collaborations. Grounding into yogic ethics and ensuring you have clear ways to communicate about what those ethics look like in practice is very helpful.

FROM "ME" TO "WE"

I think some of the best collaborations happen when the participants agree to check their egos at the door and pledge to be part of the whole. One of the most powerful—and beautiful—examples of collaborative allyship like this comes from the work of the cultural strategist and philanthropist Anasa Troutman in Memphis, Tennessee. As I understand it, her whole mission is to create a world that works for *everyone*; to create a cultural shift that can move the dial from "me" to "we." To do that, she formed a media company, a foundation, and an investment fund, which taken all together will, in Anasa's words, "revolutionize how inspiration becomes transformation."

One example of her collaborative spirit in media is the BIG We, a collective of "creative, hopeful risk-takers who are shaping culture through storytelling and strategy." Her nonprofit arts and culture foundation brings opportunities to under-resourced folks specifically focusing on women and girls, environmental wellness, and restorative economics in Southern Black communities.

Although there are definitely collaborations that feel magical and collaborations that feel like a big mismatch, there's nothing magical about creating successful collaborations that center allyship and accompliceship. Here are some suggestions to consider before you enter into a partnership—and during your time together.

Preparing to Collaborate
- Start with yourself. Make a list of the things you're good at and what you're willing to do; list tasks you're not that skilled at (or interested in) and what your boundaries are.
- What are the causes you are excited about and what kinds of collaborations are you eager to create (or join)?

- Review the yamas, which can remind you of what it means to work with others in a conscious way.
- Look for a collaborator or a group of folks who bring something to the experience that adds to what you have.

How to Be a Good Collaborator

- Understand that the whole is so much greater than the sum of its parts.
- Let go of your desire to be front and center. Place your emphasis and care on mutual uplift and a winning-together outcome.
- Help set expectations and assumptions at the very beginning, to minimize confusion.
- Prioritize and embrace diversity. An important aspect of collaboration is remembering and accepting that there are different ways to do things. Make room for all voices, experiences, and ideas.
- Remember this is about collaborating, not competing. Everyone in the group is there because they are invested in the work and working toward the same goals.
- Practice transparency, good communication skills, and clarity to support yourself, your teammates, and the greater cause that you are serving together.
- Notice how others respond emotionally to your words or actions; be empathic, open-minded, and receptive to feedback.
- Listen more than speak. Be respectful and kind in your feedback and questions, especially if you don't agree with what's being said.

Always return to your practice—on the mat and the cushion—to help ensure that you enter into any partnership or collaboration with mindful attention and the best intentions to create change on a personal, relational, and cultural level.

⣿ ALLYSHIP AND ACCOMPLICESHIP PRACTICE

- Who are your allies? What makes them allies along your journey? How do you receive their connection?
- Whose ally or accomplice have you been? What does it mean for you to be an ally or accomplice? How do you show up for others?
- What experiences or places have been allies for you in awakening?
- How can you cultivate more spiritual allyship? How can you expand your allyship and accompliceship?   ⣿

14

Trusting Your Yogic Journey

Step 7

There is something beyond our mind which abides in
silence within our mind. It is the supreme mystery beyond
thought. Let one's mind and one's subtle body rest upon
that and not rest on anything else.

—*MAITRI UPANISHAD*

OUR SADHANA PRACTICE is a constant interplay between effort
(abhyasa) and ease (vairagya). Abhyasa is all about showing up and
doing the work, and yet it also leaves room for the very human habit
of straying or drifting from our dharma when things get too hard
or we get too busy or too . . . something. It's the gentle invitation to
return to our practice, recommit to our sadhana, whenever we lose
the connection. Vairagya reminds us not to hold on too tight to what
we think should happen; to surrender to the process with openness
and curiosity. We may not always know where our practice is taking us. We may not even know why we've chosen to heed yoga's
call in the first place. But we know that by taking a leap of faith—
over and over again—and embracing the opportunity to love and be
loved, see and be seen, we surrender our need to be the savior and
pledge to serve in the true spirit of yoga—with unconditional love
and presence.

The leap-and-let-go of yoga can be a wild and immensely powerful experience. We can be going about our day, raising the kids,
doing the dishes, taking a walk, when suddenly the entire world

sparkles with light from within and we feel connected to everything. One day we are going about our work and the next day that work feels absolutely pointless and we know we are meant to live a life of conscious service. Yoga calls to us at times with a gentle voice and at times with a wildly insistent one.

Paradoxically, the more you leap, the deeper you drop down into your practice and the easier it is to receive yoga and to *be* yoga. Another paradox: the more you surrender, the more you realize you didn't lose anything in the first place. For me, the leap came in a decision I made to return to my homeland—at the risk of upsetting some of my family—so that I might understand what yoga was calling me to do.

I was born in England and raised in the United States. Similar to many immigrants, some of my family sometimes painted a picture of India that was scary, challenging, and unfavorable. Though they shared many helpful yoga practices with me, they also responded to injected oppression with a strong alliance with the dominant culture in the West. It was the only way to survive as Indian folks in a white dominant world. In one of the yoga teacher-training classes I run, my students coined the term *surthrival*—a combination of surviving and thriving. But surthrival of this sort has costs. One of the costs was a negative bias against their homeland, formed in part to survive in a world that didn't value the culture and traditions of origin. So we grew up as confused Indian children, not hearing a lot of positive things about our culture at home while the outside world was encouraging us to reject who we were for the promise of success. Everything around us affirmed white allegiance.

"Go work at your 7-Eleven." "Terrorist." "Go home." Kids on our block shouted racial epithets.

In every game we played as kids, a pattern emerged. My brother and I, the only Brown children playing on the block, had to be the bad guys—each and every game. We were the Indians. The Indians were always going to get chased, caught, lose and die. Faces shoved into the ground, the smell of concrete melting like my humiliation under the unrelenting Southern California sun with gravel digging into my resisting palms. We piled loss upon loss, gathering bruises like other kids gathered jacks or Pokémon cards. This game of persistent loss was my childhood and likely that of many others—a confusing space to be in, first as a Brown girl and then as a young woman. Luckily, I also had family members who love who they are and responded differently to systemic oppression. From them I witnessed pride, care, and connection to Indian culture.

The lullabies, visualizations, and mantras that slipped from my family's lips all started to make sense as a pathway out of self-hate and a vehicle for practice. That's when I knew I needed to go to India and study and practice more deeply. For me, this wasn't the stereotypical spiritual journey of travel to an exotic faraway destination. This was a journey of homecoming. I struggled with my decision immensely, knowing that some close family members were worried about me and didn't want me to go. Also, I had internalized a lot of fear—understandably, because every place I went, Indians and other Brown folks were feared and pushed down or pushed away. I knew I couldn't just go as a tourist; I had to stay long enough to connect with my homeland—to experience the tough times as well as the beauty and wonder.

When I stepped off the plane—despite the wild dogs, roaming cows, honking rickshaws, and the crush of beggars wanting one rupee, I got down on my knees and touched India's saffron-colored earth. Under the blazing orange sun, India's soft earth smelled of turmeric and mangoes. *I am here,* I whispered. *Welcome home,* I heard. I felt a belonging, pride, and connection that would never again be taken from me.

I had to go to India to understand my roots and myself, and more so, to understand what had happened to my culture postcolonization. It took me twenty-six years to save the money to go. This trip was not my *Eat, Pray, Love* moment. It was a lifetime of loss and memory, hope and grief, forgiveness and love. I had to take the risk of leaving everything I'd known, of disappointing those who loved me and those I loved, and follow the call. Only then could I let go of all the roadblocks I had put up to protect myself from the pain of ridicule and abuse, everything that separated me from embracing my culture. I don't believe everyone needs to take this exact journey to India like I did. This was my story and journey. We each have our unique journey. In yoga we are called to throw off illusion and seek to truly know ourselves. This invitation involves risks. Are we willing to follow the path of self-realization wherever it takes us?

⣶ LEAP-AND-LET-GO PRACTICE

- What small or big risks are you willing to take to lean into a yogic way of life? What would that look like in your day-to-day life?
- Who can support you as you explore bravery with these new leaps? Perhaps you call on an ancestor who makes you brave. This might be a land, blood, or spiritual ancestor—or even an ancestor of yoga. ⣶

BRINGING IT ALL TOGETHER

Sometimes we move yoga into our lives not so much from a leap of faith but from curiosity or a slow, steady unfolding of the practice. You may have been doing yoga for years in the privacy of your own space. You may have been in a studio setting with others on their own path of self-inquiry; moving, breathing, exploring how the ethical principles impact everyday life and wondering whether they'll help you show up in a more conscious way in your relationships and as you're called to serve. After practicing for some time, you may notice that your sadhaka practice has moved from the mat into daily life and you can see that it's affecting the ways you show up in your relationships and the ways you engage in the world. When this happens, it's a sign that you're experiencing a sense of inner and outer integration. What you're experiencing within, what you're learning about yourself, has opened your heart in a much bigger way. This integration is not a linear, step-by-step, logical process, but then nothing in yoga really is, is it? So it's helpful to think of it more as a spiral. You may have an experience one time that rocks your world and transforms your understanding of what transpired. Another time, integration may feel like a flash of realization, where everything suddenly makes sense internally *and* externally. Generally speaking, I find that inner integration is necessary for outer integration to happen. The outer integration often comes later. So it makes sense to begin with the inner.

Trusting Yourself

Embracing yoga as your spiritual practice means you are always seeking and connecting to the divine within you first before venturing outward. *Everything* is yoga for a sadhaka. There is no longer any distinction between "practice" and "living"—they are one and the same. You are now in a flow state of aligned action. To me, aligned action means being so steeped in yoga practice that I know when to act and when to be still; when to speak and when to be silent; what is in resonance with my values and what is not.

As you live with yoga, in a container of practice, full of trust and faith, it often becomes like an old friend or a part of yourself. You might start to feel that yoga is alive within you; that it has a consciousness of its own. Yoga is here with you to create more unity. This is who you've become.

You may have moments of feeling internally connected, filled up with all-in-ness, devotion with yoga. You find yourself showing up in a way that expresses that love and devotion to yoga, which is really love and devotion to yourself and everyone else. You trust: *I am going to show up for my practice and for yoga no matter what. It's who I am.*

By loving and committing in this way and being truly present, yoga gives me so much. I feel committed to honoring that and letting yoga know its value.

What does it mean to "integrate" yoga into your being? It's sometimes easier to understand how your practice can help you out there in the world—how it can enrich and inform all the ways you show up in relationship with others. (Think: the yamas, which teach us to act in ways that don't increase suffering and can help minimize separation.) Inner integration, on the other hand, is how you understand the principles of yoga from the inside—how your practice helps you treat *yourself* with kindness, make informed decisions based on the niyamas and yamas, and be more truthful about your needs, misgivings, and strengths. Beginning with internal integration can help you notice when you're not acting in integrity with your sadhana practice and provide the opportunity to course correct. From there, your practice can expand outward more readily. The inquiry becomes: *Am I in alignment or out of alignment? And what do I need to come back into my truth?*

Trust the Practice

As you bring your practice alive in the world around you and see how your friends, family (biological and chosen), colleagues, and even strangers are engaging with you in more connected ways—and you with them—you may begin to trust in the power of practice. Of course, not all relationships or situations recognize you for who you are or how you've changed—which is okay. Often those situations and relationships will drop away, quickly or over time. With those who do see the integrated you, there's often a shift in how they relate to you—and how you relate to them.

Sometimes, in our attempt to integrate more fully with others, we try too hard. We might act as if we have something to prove or that we are cooler, more spiritual, or even "better" than others. We really want others to see that we've changed, but in our attempts, we may end up alienating them instead of drawing them closer. It can be hard to recognize this stage, and we may think it's the other person's issue. Here's my suggestion (and what I do): When you do sense another person's discomfort or feel them pulling away, simply pause, do a little internal inventory, take a few calming breaths, and relax—just be yourself. Meet them where they're at and not where you want them to be.

When I was a young person, as a Brown immigrant girl I was raised to be polite and quiet. I was very shy. I struggled to make myself heard; when I spoke, no one seemed to pay attention to what I had to say. I'd be hanging out with my friends and offer an opinion or request, and it would often get ignored. I remember beginning my first teaching job in 2001 and my students literally saying, "Miss! You are teaching us, but we can't hear you!"

It was around this time that I began to turn back toward my ancestral practices of yoga and meditation more fully. I was practicing the sadhana my family and teachers had taught me, listening to talks, going to puja and practices. More than anything, I realized that in order to live according to yoga's code of ethics, I had to revisit satya and understand the importance of—and the power associated with—telling the truth. I had to own who I was. It wasn't always easy for me because when I was younger, I had become good at bending the truth, perhaps hoping that I'd sound cooler and more interesting if I embellished the facts of my life.

Nonetheless, I was devoted to my satya practice; determined to be more discerning in my speech, kinder, more committed to resolving (instead of avoiding) conflicts, even small ones; speaking up in encouraging ways. Slowly, over the course of a year, I noticed a huge change. The more comfortable I was in sharing my truth, the more confident my voice became, the more audible my delivery. My students started to listen to me, regularly attend class, do their homework, and care about school. Even my colleagues noticed. All of a sudden, I was no longer the diminutive young woman with the tiny voice that no one could hear. I was still small, but I spoke more clearly, resonantly and felt progressively more confident in the truth I had to share with my community and the world around me.

True integration—inner and outer—happens when you stop working so hard to do what's required of you or what you think you *should* do—and trust the wisdom of the practice to guide you. It doesn't mean life or relationships are perfect. Far from it. We are all human beings having a human experience! But it does mean, if we pay attention, yoga can guide us on the path and be our companion every step of the way. The more we are willing to receive what the world reflects back to us, the more we can integrate our yogic practices in our world.

⁙ TRUSTING YOURSELF PRACTICE

- What does it mean for your yoga practice to be in alignment with your values? Think of a few examples of when you felt such an integration.
- What does it mean to connect with the divine within yourself? And why is that important in a sadhaka's life?
- What does it mean to show up in a way that honors yoga's presence in your life? What are some of the ways you can do that?

Answer these reflection questions in a way that might be out of the ordinary for you: dance your answer, write, draw, sing, or invite your body to move through yoga with pure awareness and devotion. ⁙

⁙ TRUSTING THE PRACTICE

- What relationships or situations no longer feel aligned with who you are as you are embodying yoga through your life?
- Think of an experience in which you truly saw someone without any preconceived ideas or biases. And then think of an experience in which you felt someone truly saw *you* just as you are. For each experience, journal with these prompts: What did this feel like in your body? In your lungs, your heart, your belly?
- What signs of outer integration with a life of yoga do you notice in your life? ⁙

Not Too Tight, Not Too Loose

This part of the call speaks to the potency of the container. Yoga sadhana connects you to a bigger, more divine experience of self, sensuality, awareness, orienting to dharma and joy in everyday life. At this point on the sadhaka journey, it's not uncommon to feel grounded in yoga's roots, alive and healed generations back and forward. You may even experience a sense of spaciousness in which you feel connected to the sacredness of all life, one in which you remember what and who you really are. You are able to trust, live, and serve from this place. The caution here is not to become too attached to those feelings or experiences. Yoga isn't a one-and-done journey; there is no end point. We soon discover that the more we try to hold on too tightly to a feeling, an experience, or even the definition we've attached to ourselves, the more it all slips through our fingers. Yoga is a practice of exploration, development, and process—not of achievement and perfection.

Now is a good time to circle back to your practice of aparigraha—nongrasping or nonpossessiveness—and commit this mantra to memory: *Not too tight, not too loose.* Say yes to your practice. Show up from that place; use the tools in your yoga tool kit and the skills you've learned. Be okay when you fall down, when things don't go as you wanted them to or you feel like you've failed. When that happens, you begin again. Like most of us, you may need to cycle back and forth through these stages many times, even answer the call to yoga all over again. That can happen when you experience a crisis of confidence, feel the need to recommit to allyship, or reassess your relationship to a particular yoga precept. That's all normal—and beneficial. And all of that is, guess what? Yoga.

Yet there is something powerful about pausing to acknowledge and celebrate all you've already experienced, all the ways yoga has enriched your life. There is something important about reminding yourself that yoga is inherently abundant in spiritual riches. You might hold or reflect on this new vision of abundance as a living, giving, regenerative experience of life. Yoga teaches us that we are worthy of a life filled with joy, that we don't need to chase after "better" or "more than." At this stage, you simply are. There's a sense of spaciousness in which new growth can happen, new connections can arise. The twelfth-century sage Sri Adi Shankaracharya put it so beautifully:

Ever serenely balanced, I am neither free nor bound—
Consciousness and joy am I, and Bliss is where I am found.[1]

You live channeling life-force energy, full of Saraswati-like creativity, in devotion to yoga and to your community with equity. All of a sudden, you are in the midst of a yoga-pleasure revolution! There's a natural harmony that arises when one is in devotion and integrity.

There's an understanding that there's so much more than our limited smaller ego self. It's easier to let the not worthy fade away, to live from an expansive self.

In this stage, there's a play of exchange of power and energy. As you embody yoga, you are expanding into higher amounts of giving and receiving. You are moving beyond the fearful or conditioned responses.

Receive yoga and hold the energy of unity inside yourself. Open to your ability to be with higher and higher sensations of divine interconnectedness. Allow yourself to feel! When you know yoga is here, it feels safe for you to feel, breathe, and be.

This full embodiment moves forward and creates even more energy. In this state, it's often easier and easier to live and give from overflow. Everything begins to integrate.

It's what brings me joy and good in the world; what is peaceful for me in work, family, life. It feels right and good. All of this integrates into everyday life through deep yoga practice. There's a sense of interconnectedness and expansive fulfillment. Yoga is always there. You can depend upon it for fun, harmony, and uplift.

Now that we have taken our yoga from practice to embodiment, it's time to explore what it means to lead the yogic way. This type of leadership does not require that you become a yoga teacher. Many people are incredible yoga teachers or guides without ever stepping foot in front of a class or demonstrating a pose on a mat. Yoga leadership is an exciting and challenging path of continually deepening in, embodying and showing up again and again with yoga as your guide.

15

Sharing Yoga as a Sacred Practice

Step 8

When all the knots that strangle the heart are loosened,
the mortal becomes immortal, here in this very life.
—*KATHA UPANISHAD*

AS YOU PROGRESS on the sadhaka's path, you'll realize that there
is no end to your journey—that you will make a conscious commitment to yoga over and over again—and there is nothing else to do
but to serve with yoga as your guide. You'll begin to explore how
yoga can evolve to meet your needs as well as the needs of your
community and beyond.

In committing to yoga as spiritual practice, we must never forget
that yoga is a tool that can be used to heal—or to harm—and we have
choices in how we engage with it. In recent history, I think about the
work of the Dalit activist Thenmozhi Soundararajan, the author of
The Trauma of Caste, whom I mentioned in chapter 1. Soundararajan
highlights the harm that has been done to Dalit folks in the name
of yoga and how important it is to continue to address that harm
so we can turn it toward healing. Her call echoes the revolutionary
work of Dalit Buddhist leader Dr. B. R. Ambedkar—and many Indian
activists like Gaura and Sudashi Devi of the Chipko environmental movement in the 1970s and others in various liberation movements as well—in foregrounding the role their spiritual practices
played in their work for liberation and equity for all. Their values
of the essence of yoga in satyagraha, self-sovereignty, and integrity

were crucial in making challenging decisions under pressure and continuing a struggle with the sustenance and fortitude of spiritual foundations.

As sadhakas, we too must connect to the foundational ethics of yoga, which implore us to be of service for the betterment of all beings—from a place of love and truth. The same truths you tell yourself as you quiet your mind; authentic truths that come from a place of inner knowing. When we put ahimsa and satya into practice, we have essentially moved yoga deeper into our personal lives and into the world in a way that invites us—and *allows* us—to take action for our own uplift and that of others at the same time.

As we explore moving into action, we can learn from more recent freedom movements in the United States. In his 1963 letter from a Birmingham jail,[1] Dr. Martin Luther King Jr. outlines the steps for nonviolent civil disobedience inspired by the actions of those in India fighting for their freedom. He outlines, "In any nonviolent campaign there are four basic steps: collection of the facts to determine whether injustices exist; negotiation; self-purification; and direct action." All of which align with yogic principles. "Collection of the facts to determine whether injustices exists" is *vichara*, or wise discrimination. "Negotiation" is found in satya—seeing and speaking the truth with clarity and listening with an open mind. "Self-purification" is tapas, which prepares us for practice and action. Finally, "direct action" is Karma yoga, which determines how we show up in the world.

These carry forward into the "12 Steps to Changing Yourself and the World," a chapter in *An Abolitionist's Handbook*, by Patrisse Cullors, the activist and cofounder of the Black Lives Matter movement.[2] By giving us tools to help us have courageous conversations, say yes to imagination, practice accountability, allow ourselves to feel, forgive actively (not passively), Cullors invites us all to connect our spiritual and activist practices.

Moving into aligned action for me is a process of inquiring within, checking on my values, assessing my role and relationships, and deciding whether to act. I continually check back in as I move forward.

Wherever you are, you can be inspired to act. Look around you and see what is calling to you—from Earth, animals, other humans— and take action in truth. What is your satyagraha, your truth force, that you are committed to in order to relieve suffering? This is the path of an engaged yoga practitioner and steward.

✹✹ CALL TO SERVICE PRACTICE

- How is your yoga leading you to serve?
- What are the practices that support your actions of service?
- Whom can you learn from?
- How can you support others in their service?   ✹✹

PUTTING YOUR SADHANA INTO PRACTICE

Now that you know your particular leadership style, how do you put those qualities into practice? Grab a timer, a notebook, and a pen and get ready to brainstorm. Remember, don't overthink—first thought, best thought—and don't censor or judge yourself. As you write, think about your leadership style and how it relates to taking action. For each question, set a timer for five minutes and go!

- How do you want to bring your sadhana alive in the world? Consider which aspects of yoga philosophy, practices, and ethics you are most interested in exploring in your leadership.
- What is happening in the world right now that makes you feel anger or despair?
- What are you most excited about creating in the world right now?
- Why yoga? How can yoga be a powerful ally in mitigating harm?

Put your pen down and take some time to read over what you've written. You may find themes, overlaps, and even contradictions. Circle, highlight, draw lines between things that stand out or connect. And now, pick up your pen again and begin with a blank page; set the timer for five minutes for each question.

- If you could pick one issue that you're really passionate about, what would it be and why?
- If the world were more just and equitable, what would your issue look like, feel like, and be like? Feel free to draw or paint a picture of the paradise of this issue.
- How could you use yoga to address something you are really passionate about? What needs to change and how would you like to participate? An example: Challenges to reproductive rights are huge and disturbing. How could we bring yoga to support movements that demand bodily autonomy?

Tactics for Change

Remember that there are myriad ways to create change. Small and local can be just as powerful as big and worldwide! There may be things you are inspired and driven to do but you have no idea how the results will turn out. That's okay; it's not just about outcomes. It might be a soft whisper. It might be a loud roar. It might be an ask, an uplift, a dance, or a full-on revolution. Whatever it is, it's certainly a yoga changemaking dream in action!

I encourage you to take an asset-based approach to this. You don't need to pile on more obligations or learn a bunch of new skills. You can focus on something you already know how to do. Even spend some time learning more about yourself. Resilience, self-preservation, and self-care are all part of social justice. You can do what you are already doing, deepen in your practice, keep it simple.

Keeping in mind what you wrote in your brainstorming session on pages 196–97—and your elemental archetype—take a look at these seven different tactics for change. Although certainly not an exhaustive list, it'll give you some ideas of where to put your energy and how to offer your gifts of service.

1. **Direct service** means addressing people's basic needs by providing for their material well-being—food, water, shelter,

skills development, and education—as well as spiritual support, meditation, and asana. It means working directly with people to hone their ability to get what they need within the system that already exists. Some examples include providing yoga and mindfulness for specific communities, such as those who are incarcerated or housing insecure; seniors, migrants and refugees; and specific populations, such as queer, trans, and BIPOC. This is a great path for everyone and especially for empathic earth and fluid watery changemakers.

2. **Viral social / guerilla advocacy** is directly aimed at influencing the opinions or behaviors of people by delivering a specific type of message rather than impartially providing information. This can help you find your voice and get your creative juices flowing. Some examples include spoken word and songs; a zine or magazine (online or print); memes; revolutionary art (wheat-pasting public art like Robbie Conal posters); my own big events and social interventions like the Yoke Yoga social media app, Yoga Restival and the Honor {Don't Appropriate} Yoga Summit; any creative event that shares a new message that speaks to and shifts the times. This can be all the things—sexy, fun, shocking, joyful, pleasure-filled, informative, and nuanced! This type of changemaking particularly excites water, fire, and air changemakers who love fresh ideas and creativity.

3. **Political organizing** is working within the current system of power, policy, and/or government to use structures of power to create change. This could be through changing laws, redirecting funds, electing a particular candidate, or changing policy or practices. Political organizing can mean unionizing, fundraising, boycotting, lobbying your congressperson, or setting up a letter-writing campaign directed to people or organizations in power. This type of changemaking can be a powerful outlet for fire and air types who are driven and passionate.

4. **Community organizing** is getting a large number of people within a community to support a cause and then using

the power of the many to put pressure on those in power to make change. Community organizing can look like non-violent protests and marches; digital protests or campaigns (pass the mic); creating clubs or groups, such as the Black Panthers, Yogis of Color, #MeToo, Healing Circles; building yoga circles; or creating spiritual spaces/meditation spaces. This form of changemaking often involves relationship building, small or large. This is a great form of changemaking for earth-element types who are focused on steadily and methodically building power.

5. **Building alternative institutions** is a powerful way to create change by getting people's needs met outside of the existing system. Building alternative institutions can look like creating new institutions and organizations, such as NGOs, non-profits; trauma/crisis centers, like Teen Line; foundations, like Reclamation Ventures, founded by Nicole Cardoza; or programs never done before. This type of changemaking is often in the arena of air and space types who have so many powerful and revolutionary new visions and ideas.

6. **Organizing revolt** is a form of disruption using the media to forcibly make change, whether by redistributing resources, shutting down the system, or demanding a change in leadership. Organizing revolt can look like putting pressure on institutions and systems to actively catalyze change. Some examples are the Satyagraha movement for independence in India, Arab Spring, Occupy Wall Street, Yoga Teachers Walking Out, #MeToo. It can also mean boycotting institutions. This style of changemaking has to be wielded carefully to preserve ahimsa and can be incredibly powerful for fire and air changemakers.

7. **Spiritual changemaking** works by sharing parables and stories and through living a life of spiritual principles dedicated to shaping change. A compelling example of spiritual changemaking comes out of South Central Los Angeles and the work of the longtime spiritual activist and cultural creator Eisha Mason, who believes in—and is driven by—the

restorative power of justice, equity, creativity, imagination, nonviolence and love. I met Eisha Mason when she taught a class on nonviolence for peacemakers. She introduced me to the work of Thich Nhat Hanh and has supported me and so many others in continuing our work over the decades. Good friends with Reverend James Lawson from civil rights activism, Mason brings the power of spiritual changemaking alive in everything she does—whether working as executive director of the American Friends Service Council or leading sermons and classes with Agape Spiritual Center; or in her work of storytelling, community building, and supporting BIPOC, environmental wellness, and social change. No matter what the project is, spirit is at the heart of it for Mason. Spiritual changemakers like Mason and so many others are driven by a clear sense of our interconnection and draw their power into protecting that interbeing however they can. The space archetype is most powerfully aligned to this form of changemaking.

Teaching Yoga as Sacred Practice

As yoga stewards, we have heeded the call and chosen to walk the path of a yoga sadhaka. We've been steeped in the practice that we love—we study it, we practice it, we live it—and we're committed to sharing it with others, knowing yoga's ability to transform lives both individually and communally. Many of us choose to share yoga's gifts by becoming yoga teachers, presenting the practices in an accessible way through the qualities we embody and the skills we have learned. Our teaching becomes an extension of our sadhana, our inner spiritual practice.

In order to truly teach, you must cultivate a deeply personal relationship with all aspects of the practice. That means you allow asana and pranayama to take their rightful place within the eight limbs of yoga, not any more important than the yamas, niyamas, and the inward-directed practices of concentration, meditation, and union with the divine. That means you consider carefully which aspects of yoga you are willing and able to share and which ones you keep as part of your own sacred practice. You take into account cultural and political issues, being mindful around cultural appropriation, inclusion, and diversity. You ensure that you practice spiritual lineage acknowledgment and let students know the richness of the full yoga tradition, even if you are not sharing all aspects of it. Ideally, all yoga teachers should be devoted student-stewards of yoga.

Before we dive into what yoga leadership looks like in yoga studio and classroom spaces, let's consider the way we often use the term *yogi* or *yogini*, as in *I am a yogini* or *They are true yogis*. I've never been comfortable calling myself that, or having someone else refer to me as a "yogi" or "yogini." Don't get me wrong—to be a yoga teacher is an incredible honor. We are so fortunate to be able to explore, live, and embody a sacred wisdom practice, one that has worked for thousands of years to reduce suffering and increase compassionate connection and peace. And then through our very being and our words, we get to pass it along to others as authentically as we can.

However, being a yoga teacher doesn't mean we are yogis. In India, *yogi* is someone who has renounced all attachment to the external world and has given their entire life in practice for moksha, or liberation. Even Henry David Thoreau of Walden Pond fame, who chose to live in a simple outdoor dwelling by a pond for a time and often questioned the purpose of life, studied the sacred Vedic texts. He understood the tenuous nature of being a yogi. He famously said, "Even I, at times, am a yogi." He instinctively knew that "yogi" wasn't a label to be thrown around lightly but a profound state or experience of liberation and detachment from the conventional concerns of the mundane everyday world.

RESPONSIBILITIES OF A YOGA TEACHER

So, for those of us who are not already enlightened yogis, the label "yoga teacher" or "yoga steward" feels just right. It's an intimate and powerful position to be in—one we must never abuse or take for granted. How we share what yoga is can help our students get more in touch with their own bodies, their own breath, and their own

202 HEEDING THE SADHAKA'S CALL

freedom. We get to provide space for people to experience yoga in a way that honors its roots; in a way that ensures that the practice is accessible to all and not dependent on anyone's physical ability, skill level, or social location. A space in which they can begin to strip away the conditioning of capitalism, patriarchy, and consumerism and perhaps experience what it feels like to honor and love themselves in a more holistic way and, in doing so, love and work for the liberation of others.

As my teacher Shankarji used to jokingly and lovingly point out to me when I felt really accomplished or had really understood something, "Ha, ha—you think you know so much! You could study yoga your whole lifetime and still barely scratch the surface!" His words have kept me humble in my role as teacher and reinforced my commitment to continual learning.

On a practical level, what are some of the responsibilities of a yoga teacher? Consider the list below and feel free to add your own bullet points.

- **Maintain a personal practice.** This is essential. You can't teach what you don't know, and you can't know what you don't live.
- **Honor the sacredness of your personal yoga practice** and ask yourself such questions as *What am I leading or inviting others to do? How can this practice bring more self-awareness and foster more self-love and love for others?*
- **Be a perennial student of yoga.** Never forget that you are a student first, and keep the yogic flame burning (for yourself and others).
- **Listen deeply**—to your students and your own inquiry. Listen for the question underneath the words being spoken.
- **Create a space in which everyone feels welcome, safe, and supported,** no matter what type of yoga you teach.
- **Hold space for other people to create change for themselves.** But always remember we can never know another's experience. It's theirs to have. We are merely guides and they are the leaders.

- **Teach with clarity, confidence, and compassion.** No matter what you're teaching, the golden rule of yoga is always to do no harm.

FINDING YOUR VOICE

Finding your voice (or rediscovering it) as a yoga teacher is really no different from finding it within your relationships or in your commitment to service. It's an inward exploration that is part of what it means to create sovereignty for self and others. When we feel clear and confident in our offerings, our voice reflects that. Of course, the opposite is true as well. When we feel tentative, less than sure of our knowledge or our ability to impart it, or simply out of our element, doing something we've not ever done before, our voice can falter and get very small.

I had such an experience not that long ago as I was preparing to deliver my TEDx Talk, "How Speaking Your Truth Can Spark a Movement."[3] I had a crisis of confidence and was racked with doubt and insecurities even though I had spoken and written about that topic countless times before. Despite months of preparation and a deep desire to share, I seriously considered pulling the plug. I care so much about the message of honoring the roots of yoga and I wanted to do my ancestors proud. But each time I practiced, it just wasn't working. I felt tight and insecure. My throat closed and my movements felt stiff and awkward. I was having full-body shakes and so much mental chatter and anxiety. These are familiar reactions for me, a person who's been shy for much of my life.

Thankfully, yoga has tools to deal with physical manifestations and intrusive thoughts like these. So I took a break from practicing my talk and instead turned back to practicing my yoga. I did asana, chanted, meditated, and read the sacred texts that had always comforted me. I napped and rested my conscious and subconscious mind in yoga nidra. It worked. With the support of my practice, I returned to my TEDx Talk with renewed confidence. When my turn came to speak, I nailed it! I spoke from my heart and I felt that I made my teachers, family, and ancestors proud.

Overall, as challenging as this experience was, I'm glad I persevered. The irony, of course, was that my talk was about speaking up even in the places where you feel most insecure and how doing so could quite possibly be the key to changing a broken system and changing yourself. And I had almost failed to heed my own advice!

It doesn't matter how long you've been doing this work—you can still suffer a momentary crisis of confidence. However it happens that you lose your voice or struggle to find your way into the practice or teaching, know that you're not alone. You can turn to mentors, colleagues, and friends for guidance. You can return to your practice and draw upon its wellspring of nourishment for strength. You've got this! And we've got you!

⠿ Reflections on Finding Your Voice

Here are a few questions to ponder as you explore how best to share your gifts with the world.

- What is something really important to you that you don't speak or write about enough?
- What is on your heart that you are afraid to share but matters deeply to you?
- Around whom or in what environments do you feel more like yourself and what environments make you feel smaller? How can you play with the energy of expansion and contraction and expand even in spaces that might normally make you feel like contracting?
- What physical movements can support your vocal expression?
- What phrases, affirmations, or mantras could you use to help unlock your voice?   ⠿

Preserving the Tradition

As you live within a container of practice, full of trust and faith, yoga becomes like an old friend or a deep part of yourself. You connect to yoga as a way of yoking all the things that have become separate within you. Even as you do that in your personal practice, it can be hard sometimes to know how to share that when you're teaching others. I'm often asked, "How can I teach asana as a spiritual practice, one that honors yoga's roots?"

I know it can be hard to imagine that's even possible here in the West where yoga is part of fitness culture. That's because we've been led to believe people *want* that yoga body they see on social media—flexible, lithe, and strong—which is nothing but a construct based on dominant culture. Even if teachers are well versed in the true fundamentals of yoga, they may find it difficult to attract students (or make a living, if that is a goal) without minimizing the spiritual aspects and resorting to gimmicks like goat yoga, cacao yoga, or happy hour yoga. It can all feel so discouraging and overwhelming. Even more important: not aligning with the principles of yoga is antithetical to the heart of this ancient practice. We can aim to do no harm and to create spaces of inclusion and union by offering trauma-informed yoga and creating truly accessible classes.

The most powerful way to preserve the tradition in your teaching, as we've talked about a lot in this book, is to study, practice, and bring it into your own life. It means naming and honoring yoga's roots, including more of what the full expanse of this practice is: mantra, mudra, meditation, pranayama, philosophy, and more yogic depth. You can practice, live, teach, and share yoga beyond asana. It also means when you teach yoga asana, you present it in a way that honors the sacredness of the physical body, moving through poses intentionally and lovingly as a way of getting to know ourselves a little bit better. Asana, after all, is an integral part of the spiritual practice of yoga.

How do we facilitate that as teachers who are stewarding this sacred tradition? How do we infuse our asana teaching with yoga philosophy? Above all, we do this by bringing our own experiences with the practice—our own curiosity—into our teaching and honoring the students we teach. Through our very being and teaching we are passing along and nourishing this true gift to the world as authentically as possible. On a practical level, one way to do this is to create a structure that weaves yoga philosophy into our sequencing. Here's a framework I use in many of my classes:

1. I begin by choosing a practice, yogic tenet, or element that I've been working with for a long time.

2. Once I feel like I am in relationship to this teaching, I choose a theme for the class. It could be a message or a shloka—a verse or a phrase that we can play with in movement and breathing techniques; or I choose one of the eight limbs.

3. Then I build a sequence that invites students to investigate the theme in their bodies and lives, to move deeper into self-inquiry, exploring what it means to connect with themselves. And then I ask them questions to bring them deeper into their own autonomy and awareness: "Is this shape creating space in your body? What is your body saying in this pose? What is your breath saying in this shape? Is there anything that feels "off" about this pose? Can you feel the joy within this pose? How are you feeling?"

4. I like to cue in ways that create space for students to be aware of their own presence. So they tune in to whatever they are feeling. They can get present to feel the grief, joy, numbness, and peace in their body—to feel what is truly there.

5. I think about how to move from a precise alignment-based focus to one that allows for individual autonomy and moves from a purely physical to a sense of deep spiritual inquiry.

6. For me, a part of the journey as a teacher is to bring in the quality of student-centered autonomy and empowerment. This is part of yoga as a spiritual journey. As a teacher and practitioner, I've experienced my own connection and autonomy with yoga.

7. As B. K. S. Iyengar says, "If you aren't feeling joy, you aren't practicing yoga!" I guide us into practicing and loosening that grip of what it means to practice. Yoga does help me be strong, serene, and balanced—and not just on a physical level.

If you'd like to take a short, complimentary masterclass with me that gives you a sequence, and shows you how I incorporate yoga philosophy into my teaching and how you can too, please visit IgniteYourYoga.com.

Spiritual Connection through Our Stories

I love to bring the deeper teachings into my classes in creative ways. One way I do that is by teaching asana as a form of storytelling. Try sharing your story, the story of yoga, and how it shows up in your daily life—and invite your students into their own story. Where does yoga live within those stories? How does it show up in their bodies and minds? After all, our lives begin and end with stories.

Everything in our lives is filtered through spiritual practice and possibility. This is another reason for centering our stories in our hearts as we practice. I believe by doing so, we can help tell new, liberatory stories and mitigate the harm caused by fundamentalism or colonization of yoga. Maybe you or your students' ancestors were silenced, forbidden to tell their stories, run businesses, worship freely, or live the lives they wanted. Rather than be silenced, our stories are here to be spoken and shared. We can imagine a different future when we move into it together. By bringing stories into our bodies in movement and ritual, we give voice to the stories of others, along with our own. In this way, we can perhaps ease suffering, reposition yoga as a sacred practice available to everyone, and hopefully stop intergenerational trauma from going forward to future generations. Yoga invites us into a generative way of being where we move inside the stories of the future we are creating together. Yoga is a deeply spiritual practice inviting us toward our own and others' liberation, creating a virtuous cycle of truth and uplift with yoga as unity.

⁘ REFLECTION QUESTIONS FOR SHARING YOGA

- When you step on the mat or when you're out in the world, how can your yoga still be a spiritual practice?

- How is being a yoga teacher part of your dharma? What does it look like in your own life?
- What stories, perhaps from the yoga tradition, are you curious about—that you might not know and can learn?
- What are some of your stories—and the stories of your ancestors—you wish to tell?   ⁞⁞

We've traveled together on a journey through the foundations of a full, expansive yoga practice and explored how these foundations show up in our relationships and everyday lives as well as our leadership. We've looked at social-change tactics that we can explore with yoga's support to make the world a better place, and found rich explorations and inquiries to bring soul and spirit alive in our practice and our world.

No matter what we read or what I write, this is a spiritual journey where all that matters is what we put into practice. This book and work are here to support you. You have what you need to move in the world as a yoga steward. To come back to yogic ethics when in doubt as you grow your leadership. To surrender your will and control into oneness as you practice presence. To allow yoga to move through you as you live yoga as a sacred act. Giving it all away as you serve and make change in the world with yoga as your guide.

SADHAKAS SPEAK: LINDA SPARROWE

⁞⁞

As I move into my seventies, I have come to realize that there is no separation between my spiritual practice and my daily life; between my work in the world and my dharma. Every connection I make, every experience I have—the sweetest ones as well as the hardest ones—is an opportunity to show up fully with as much friendliness, compassion, and patience as I can. Of course I don't always succeed; in fact, sometimes I fail miserably. However, when I commit to my practice of deep listening, I remember that we all long to connect, we all want to be heard. And that's when I know that my dharma is to partner with others to draw out those stories and do whatever I can to amplify them. Having said all that, what really allows me to live my spiritual practice is to receive and give unconditional love—as a grandmother. There's seriously nothing like it!

—Linda Sparrowe, longtime yoga teacher,
mentor, and author

Note to Reader

Sadhakas Speak: You

Dear Reader,

Thank you for going on this spiritual journey, a deep practice of embodiment and leadership in yoga. Now I'd love to hear from you.

How are you practicing, living, and leading as a yoga sadhaka? Please take some time to write your truth.

And if you are willing, share with art, poetry, practices, affirmations, or invocations.

You are never alone. We are a powerful community of yoga stewards! Let's create a living art wall of all the yoga sadhakas who generously live, practice, and share their journey. You inspire me, and we inspire one another.

Please share your words, images, and reflections on your journey in the yoga sadhaka space I've created for us at IgniteYourYoga.com.

Epilogue: A Prayer of Interconnection

I'm sitting at my kitchen table and staring into a candle I lit for you. I watch the flickering flame, the same in my candle as yours. Same as in the sacred fires that burn in the foothills of the Himalayas, where sannyasins practiced for thousands of years. I see in the ever-changing flame our absolute interconnection.

Now, I am no fully baked yoga muffin of an enlightened being. But all of my greatest teachers—some of whom are pretty much mostly baked—proclaim it is a continued practice of love grounded in yoga ethics. I feel this has got to be the kind of love that arises when you are not just equal to the other but you see yourself in them; when you aren't putting yourself above or below someone but truly feeling and being with them.

It's been in heartfelt connections that I've learned this yogic love. I've learned so much. I've grown. I've tried and failed, listened and learned, and tried again. I've loved being with and alongside you. Yoga is a spiritual journey that transforms me as I work to offer service with love to the world. As one moment ends and another begins, I feel a commitment to stare deep into the flame of yogic wisdom and continue to do my best to honor yoga's roots alongside those who also wish to do so.

I'm so grateful to be walking this path, following the light, here with you.

Closing Invocation

लोकाः समस्ताः सुखिनो भवन्तु
OM LOKĀH: SAMASTĀH: SUKHINO BHAVANTU

May all beings in all realms be free from suffering,
be safe, happy, and experience everlasting peace.

Glossary

This glossary gives simple definitions of working terms used in the book. It is not exhaustive but gives brief definitions of concepts and terms. It is an invitation to continue to research and learn more.

aap tattva: Water element.

abhyanga: Ayurvedic practice of self-care and massage with warmed oil.

abhyasa: Consistent effort. Often paired with the letting go of vairagya.

accessibility: Refers to the design of products, devices, services, or environments to be accessed for people who experience disabilities.

accomplice: Someone who uses their privilege to address and dismantle systems of oppression.

Adivasi: A member or descendant of the Indigenous peoples of South Asia.

Advaita Vedanta: Nondual form of yoga and Hinduism. Belief in interconnection, oneness, and unity of all things.

agni tattva: Fire element.

ahamkara: "I-ness." Identification of self.

ahimsa: Non-harm, kindness.

aita: Grandmother.

Ajivikas: A member of a nontheistic religious sect resembling Jainism, founded by Maskarin Gosala, a Buddha contemporary.

akash tattva: Space element.

ally: Someone who advocates for and supports members of a community other than their own, reaching across differences to achieve mutual goals.

allyship: A practice of active support for the rights of a marginalized or underestimated group, without being a member of that group.

aparigraha: Letting go; nonattachment.

asana: Seat, posture. The physical practice of yoga postures.

ascetics: Those who practice severe self-discipline and abstention from indulgences.

ashrama: Stage of life. The traditional Vedic stages of life are student, householder, forest dweller, renunciate.

asteya: Non-stealing, generosity.

AUM: Sacred sound.

austerity: Renunciation or giving up; a tapas practice.

Ayurveda: A system of healing and wellness that originated in India. This ancient Indian science of well-being comes from *ayuh*, meaning "life" or "longevity," and *veda*, meaning "study of."

Bhagavad Gita: A seven-hundred-verse Sanskrit scripture and a foundational text of yogic knowledge and wisdom.

bhumis (citta bhumis): Five states of mind described in the Sutras. *Kshipta bhumi*, is the disturbed, restless, distracted mind—monkey mind. *Mudha bhumi* is the dull, lethargic, sleepy, what's-the-point mind that is often accompanied by depression and sadness. *Vikshipta bhumi* is the partially focused mind, which has moments of clarity and concentration but gets pulled away easily. *Ekagra bhumi* is the single-pointed mind, which is fully focused on the object it has chosen. *Niruddha,* is the state in which the fluctuations of the mind have been stilled and the mind is in a state of pure awareness.

BIPOC: Black, Indigenous, (and) People of Color.

brahmacharya: Awareness of the divine; constraint of energy.

Brahman: This term generally refers to ideas, practices, or traditions associated with *Brahmanism*, an ancient religious tradition that was the precursor to Hinduism. It is rooted in the Vedic texts and emphasizes the worship of Brahman, the ultimate reality or universal spirit in Hindu philosophy. It can also refer to the broad cultural religious and philosophical practices tied to the Vedic system beyond the caste system.

Brahminical: Of or pertaining to the Brahmin caste.

Brahminical patriarchy: Pertaining to the power structure created for male and Brahmin caste.

brahmaviharas: The Buddhist practice of loving-kindness, compassion, empathy, and equanimity.

burnout: Chronic persistent stress that leads to overwhelm and reduces functioning.

caste: A system of oppression; a fixed social group into which an individual is supposedly born; a system of social stratification.

colonialism: System of oppression fulfilled by controlling a country, occupying it, settling it, and exploiting its natural resources and cultural and Indigenous wealth.

cultural appropriation: Taking something from a culture that is not one's own. Involves privilege and a power imbalance plus harm to the source culture and its people. The harm can be of disrespect as well as material, cultural, financial, economic, social, and spiritual harm.

Dalit: Translates to "broken"; the caste called untouchable. But as Thenmozhi Soundararajan explains in her book, *Dalit* also represents the resilience, survival, and the pride of Dalit people.

decolonization: Working to restore the original ownership of the land and resources from those from whom they have been taken or stolen. Also used to refer to a process of undoing the mindset of being colonized.

dehumanize: To make a person seem less human in order to justify mistreatment.

Desis: Diasporic Indians who live outside India.

Dharana: Mindfulness and focus.

dharma: Purpose, law, divine order.

dhyana: Meditation.

discrimination: The unjust treatment and acting out of prejudice in a way that harms a person or group based on identity, such as race, class, gender identity, sexual expression, and so forth.

diversity: Respecting, including, and celebrating differences. These can be along the dimensions of race, ethnicity, gender, sexual orientation, socioeconomic status, age, physical abilities, religious beliefs, political beliefs, or other identifying factors.

drishti: Focus and steadiness of the gaze.

East Asians: People who are from China, Korea, Japan, Taiwan, Tibet, or Mongolia.

Ebo ceremony: African spiritual ritual often involving a sacrifice.

ekagraha **bhumi:** Single-pointed focus, an essential yogic technique used to quiet the mind.

epistemology: The study of what we know and how we know it.

equity: Giving everyone what they need to be successful, taking into account the vast diversity of structural privilege, power, oppression, and life experience. Equity identifies and strives to eliminate blocks that have prevented some groups or people from participating fully.

Gayatri Mantra: A sacred mantra from the *Rig Veda*.

grihastha: Householder.

guru: A respected or esteemed teacher usually who holds a position in a teaching lineage.

guru-shishya: Guru lineage passed from teacher to student.

Hatha Yoga Pradipika: Yogic text describing the spiritual path of development while practicing yoga.

healing justice: A movement led by BIPOC people that acknowledges the healing tools and power of our ancestors and acknowledges that our illnesses or maladies are not individual events but are socially created, so healing and the creation of wellness must take into account justice.

heteronormativity: A prejudiced belief based on the gender binary that heterosexuality is the typical or normal orientation.

inclusion: An intention or policy of including people who might otherwise be excluded or marginalized, such as those who are handicapped or learning disabled, or racial and sexual minorities.

Indigenous: Native to a place, people or practice.

institutional oppression: Arrangement of a society used to benefit one group at the expense of another through the use of language, media, education, religion, economics, and the like.

internalized oppression: The result and process by which an oppressed person comes to believe, accept, or live out the inaccurate stereotypes and misinformation about their group.

kalyanamitra: Spiritual friend.

karma: Action, taking personal responsibility; fate.

karma yoga: School of yoga that focuses on action.

karuna: Compassion.

kheer: Sweet rice pudding.

kishvara pranidhana: Devotion to the divine and study of sacred texts.

koshas: Energetic sheaths described in the Upanishads, including annamaya kosha, your physical body; pranamaya kosha, your breath body; manomaya kosha, your thinking mind; vijnanamaya kosha, your wisdom body; and anandamaya kosha, your bliss body.

lila: Humor and play. Taking delight in the present moment as well as the eternal play of god or the divine. Divine love.

lineage: Where a student has learned their yogic knowledge.

maitri: Loving-kindness. *Metta* in Pali.

mantra: Sacred sound. A word or phrase repeated consistently to support the mind and aid focus.

mantra japa: Repetition of sacred sound intended to calm the mind.

metta: Pali word for loving-kindness.

moksha: Liberation.

mudita: Joyful uplift. Sympathetic joy.

mudra: Sacred gesture.

niyamas: Inner yogic codes.

oppression: Political, economic, social, cultural putting-down of people, groups, or individuals.

pagan ritual: Earth-based rituals and celebrations.

Pali: Indo-Aryan language of Theravadan Buddhism.

Patanjali: A second-third century sage who is credited with codifying and writing the Yoga Sutras.

power: The ability to affect one's will on the world and create change.

power over: External power to control, dominate, or enact one's will over another.

pranayama: Breath and life force.

pranic: From the Sanskrit word *prana* meaning "vital life force."

pratyahara: Letting go.

prejudice: A prejudgment about someone or something based on assumptions.

prithvi tattva: Earth element.

privilege: Unearned advantages.

puja: Ceremonial worship. Making an offering to the divine.

race: Classifications used to group human beings because of shared physical traits, such as skin color.

racism: (Discrimination + power) Any attitude, action, or practice backed up by institutional power that harms people because they belong to a particular racial group; a system of social, economic, political, or other advantage/privilege bestowed on people who possess certain physical trait(s).

Raja Yoga: Kingly yoga, or complete yoga.

renunciate: One who gives up the pleasures of the world in order to focus on spiritual growth and attainment.

reparations: Atoning for what has been stolen and returning many of the benefits, rights, and profits of a culture's inheritance to its creators and culture.

resource: Anything that creates a sense of internal safety, enabling us to explore, unpack, and make sense of a past experience.

sadhaka: An agent of spiritual possibility. Someone who follows a spiritual way of life designed to realize one's ideal goal.

sadhana: Individual inner spiritual practice.

samadhi: Bliss, liberation.

samanya dharma: The moral and ethical codes that apply to everyone, which are outlined in the yamas and niyamas.

sama vritti: Equal breathing practice.

samskaras: Our ingrained habits and patterns.

samyama: The combined practice of dharana (mindfulness), dhyana (concentration), and samadhi (bliss), otherwise known as insight states accessible during meditation.

sanatana dharma: The eternal and unchanging nature of the universe.

sankalpa: Deep, heartfelt, soul-level intention.

sannyasin: A renunciate who casts aside worldly concerns of money, stature, or comfort in pursuit of spiritual aims, usually in yogic tradition.

Sanskrit: Ancient Indo-European language of India used to write the Hindu scriptures and classical Indian poems.

santosha: Joy.

satya: Truth.

satyagraha: Truth force. This can be both a movement and a concept/practice.

saucha: Keeping one's mind and body pure and clean.

savasana: Corpse pose.

seva: Service and devotion.

Shakti: Life force, power.

Shankaracharya: A twelfth-century Vedic scholar from India who revived Hinduism, taught in a nondual Advaita Vendanta way; his tradition aimed at critical thinking and dispelling doubt, confusion, and ignorance.

Shankarji: The author's own spiritual teacher.

shloka: A verse or phrase that may be chosen as a theme for a yoga class.

Siddhartha Gautama: Enlightened person and teacher from second century C.E. known as the Buddha.

South Asians: People who are from Afghanistan, Pakistan, India, Bangladesh, Nepal, Bhutan, Sri Lanka, or Maldives.

Southeast Asians: Come from countries that are south of China, east of India. This includes eleven countries: Thailand, Vietnam, Malaysia, Singapore, the Philippines, Laos, Indonesia, Brunei, Burma (Myanmar), Cambodia, and East Timor.

spiritual lineage acknowledgment: Making an effort to name and acknowledge the spiritual roots of the practice of yoga in India as well as naming one's teachers.

sramana: Seeker of an austere path to spiritual freedom, rejecting the authority of the Brahmins.

Sri Adi Shankaracharya (also Adi Shankara): An Indian teacher and saint from the eighth century C.E. who helped revive Advaita Vedanta and spread yogic teachings through a system of monasteries.

stereotype: A belief about a group that doesn't take individual differences into account.

sterilization: A form of cultural appropriation that occurs when one sanitizes the practice by taking out the cultural elements of the practice to make it more palatable to the dominant culture.

sthira: Steadiness.

sukha: Ease.

svadharma: Personal dharma or purpose. How you choose to live your most conscious life.

svadhyaya: Self-inquiry.

Swami: Spiritual practitioner or teacher.

systemic oppression: The political, economic, social, cultural putting-down of people, groups, or individuals.

tapas: Yogic discipline and austerity practice.

tattva **element**: See the five elements: *prithvi, aap, agni, vayu,* and *akash*.

trauma: Anything overwhelming that impacts the nervous system in a way in which we are unable to cope or respond and causes fragmentation in mind-body-spirit.

Upanishad: Sitting at the feet of a sage or teacher. Sacred texts from the Vedic tradition.

upeksha: Equanimity, nonattachment.

using privilege: Leveraging privilege to uplift others.

vairagya: Ease, surrender.

vanaprastha: Forest dweller, retiree.

vasanas: Our subconscious tendencies.

vayu tattva: Air element.

Veda: Ancient Sanskrit texts.

Vedic meditation: Meditation based on practices found in Vedic texts, such as AUM or visualizations.

vichara: Self-inquiry, wise discrimination.

vishesha dharma: A specific duty.

white: People whose origins come from Europe.

white supremacy: A system of power that privileges white people and posits that white people are fundamentally superior, better, more intelligent than other people. The belief that white people are superior to all other races and that they should therefore hold the highest positions in society and dominate all other races.

yamas: Yoga ethics.

yamas and niyamas: Ethical foundations of yoga. They represent a yogic vision for a global yoga practice, lifestyle, and ethic.

yoga: A spiritual practice that originated in South Asia. The Sanskrit word *yoga* describes both a state of the union, oneness, or connection in consciousness and experience and the techniques, philosophies, practices, and lifestyle that bring one to such a state. The development, codification, and practice aimed at engendering oneness we understand as yoga has been practiced, cultivated, and explored over time, particularly on the Indian subcontinent, for thousands of years. Today, what we understand as yoga explores this interconnected state of consciousness, along with the development of physical health, emotional regulation, and well-being.

yoga nidra: Yogic relaxation and rest.

yoga sadhana: Deep, committed yoga practice; the deepening of these many and varied practices.

Yoga Sutras: One of the foundational texts of yoga, attributed to Sage Patanjali, codified and written in the second century B.C.E.

Yoga Vashistha: An influential sixth-century C.E. spiritual text containing elements of Hinduism and all the Shramanic traditions.

yogi/yogini: A realized master in yoga.

YTT 300: Advanced yoga teacher training (300 hours).

yuj: Union.

Notes

BEGINNING INVOCATION

1. Eknath Easwaran, trans., *"Taittiriya Upanishad* 2.2.2," in *The Upanishads* (Tomales, CA: Nilgiri Press, 2007): 115–16.

1. YOGA STEWARDSHIP

1. Thenmozhi Soundararajan, *The Trauma of Caste: A Dalit Feminist Meditation on Survivorship, Healing, and Abolition* (Oakland, CA.: North Atlantic Books, 2022): 80.
2. Pandit Rajmani Tigunait, *Secrets of the Yoga Sutra: Samadhi Pada* (Honesdale, PA: Himalayan Institute Press, 2007).

2. THE YAMAS

1. Martin Luther King Jr., "The Other America" (speech, Stanford University, April 14, 1967).
2. M. K. Gandhi, *From Yeravda Mandir* (Ahmedabad, India: Jitendra T. Desai / Navajivan Publishing House, 1936).
3. Swami Nityaswarupananda, trans., *Ashtavakra Gita: The Song of Self Knowledge* (Rishikesh: Advaita Ashrama, 2014).
4. B. K. S. Iyengar, *Light on Life: The Yoga Journey to Wholeness, Inner Peace, and Ultimate Freedom* (New York: Rodale Books, 2005): 199.

3. THE NIYAMAS

1. B. K. S. Iyengar, *Light on Yoga: Yoga Dipika* (New York: Schocken Books, 1979).
2. Pandit Rajmani Tigunait, "How to Live a Truly Joyful Life," *Yoga International*, accessed March 29, 2024.
3. Sheena Sood, "Cultivating a Yogic Theology of Collective Healing: A Yogini's Journey Disrupting White Supremacy, Hindu Fundamentalism, and Casteism," *Yoga and Race Journal*, March 2017.

4. ASANA, PRANAYAMA AND PRATYAHARA

1. Swami Vivekananda, "Addresses at The Parliament of Religions," in *The Complete Works of Swami Vivekananda*, vol. 1 (Calcutta: Advaita Ashrama, 1989). Originally presented at the World's Parliament of Religions, Chicago, September 1893.
2. David Frawley, "Pratyahara: Yoga's Forgotten Limb," *Yoga International*, accessed April 20, 2024, https://yogainternational.com/article/view/pratyahara-yogas-forgotten-limb/.

5. DHARANA, DHYANA, AND SAMADHI

1. Nischala Joy Devi, *The Secret Power of Yoga: A Woman's Guide to the Heart and Spirit of the Yoga Sutras* (New York: Harmony Books, 2007).
2. Ram Jain, "Understanding Patanjali's 5 States of Mind and How to Master the Meditative State," Arhanta Yoga, June 25, 2024, www.arhantayoga.org/blog/patanjalis-5-states-of-mind/; and "Five Chittas of Human Consciousness," Nepal Yoga Home, accessed October 1, 2023, https://nepal yogahome.com/five-chittas-human-consciousness.
3. Pandit Rajmani Tigunait, *Patanjali's Yoga Sutras* (Honesdale, PA: Himalayan Institute Press, 2014).

6. BECOMING AN AGENT OF SPIRITUAL POSSIBILITY

1. Joseph Campbell, *The Hero with a Thousand Faces* (Princeton, NJ: Princeton University Press, 1949).
2. Indu Arora, "For Your Soul: Sankalpa—a Promise to Yourself," Yoga Sadhna, January 7, 2021, www.yogsadhna.com/library/for_your_soul/sankalpa_-_a_promise_to_yourself_.
3. "The Four Brahmaviharas?" *Lion's Roar*, November 19, 2019, www.lionsroar.com/buddhism/four-divine-abodes-brahmaviharas.
4. Thanissaro Bhikkhu, "The Brahma-viharas: Head and Heart Together," *Tricycle*, Summer 2009, tricycle.org/magazine/head-heart-together/.

7. THE FOUR STAGES OF SADHANA

1. Salina Yoon, *Penguin and Pinecone: A Friendship Story* (New York: Bloomsbury, 2023).

8. EMBRACING THE CALL TO YOGA

1. I explore social location more in depth in my book *Embrace Yoga's Roots: Courageous Ways to Deepen Your Practice* (Los Angeles: Ignite Yoga & Wellness Institute, 2020).
2. Eve Tuck and K. Wayne Yang, "Decolonization Is Not a Metaphor," *Semantic Scholar*, September 8, 2012, www.semanticscholar.org/paper/Decolonization-is-not-a-metaphor-Tuck-Yang/9e908da74710e.

10. Honoring Relationships

1. Rolf Sovik, "Yoga and the Ego," Yoga International, accessed November 8, 2023, yogainternational.com/article/view/yoga-and-the-ego.

11. Moving Into Conscious Leadership

1. "The True Meaning of Dharma," Vipassana Research Institute, accessed January 20, 2024, www.vridhamma.org/discourses/The-True-Meaning-of -Dharma.

2. Quoted in Emilie Pelletier, "How to Live Your Dharma: True Purpose and the Path to Soul-Level Fulfillment," Tiny Buddha, accessed January 12, 2024, https://tinybuddha.com/blog/how-to-live-your-dharma-true-purpose -the-path-to-soul-level-fulfillment.

12. Self-Care as We Serve

1. "Burnout," Psychology Today, accessed February 15, 2024, www.psychology today.com/us/basics/burnout.

2. Audre Lorde, "Learning From the 60s," in *Sister Outsider: Essays and Speeches* (Berkeley, CA: Crossing Press, 2007): 138.

3. Audre Lorde, *A Burst of Light: And Other Essays* (Mineola, NY: Ixia Press, 2017): front flap.

4. Anana Johari Harris Parris, *Self Care Matters: A Revolutionary Approach* (Self Care Agency, 2016).

13. Collaborating with Allies on the Path

1. Jonathan Osler, "Opportunities for White People in the Fight for Racial Justice," White Accomplices, accessed October 1, 2023, www.whiteaccom plices.org.

14. Trusting Your Yogic Journey

1. Pandit S. Subrahmanya Sastri and T. R. Srinivasa Ayyangar, *Saundarya Lahari (The Ocean of Beauty) of Sri Sankara Bhagavatapada* (Madras, India: Theosophical Publishing House, 1948).

15. Sharing Yoga as a Sacred Practice

1. Martin Luther King Jr., "Letter from Birmingham Jail," Southern Christian Leadership Conference, 1963, UPenn, www.africa.upenn.edu/Articles _Gen/Letter_Birmingham.html.

2. Patrisse Cullors, *An Abolitionist's Handbook: 12 Steps to Changing Yourself and the World* (New York: St. Martin's Press, 2022).

3. Susanna Barkataki, "How Speaking Your Truth Can Spark a Move-ment," TEDx Delthorne Women, December 6, 2022. www.youtube.com /watch?v=T37-I8A6iXY.

Bibliography

Akers, Brian Dana, trans. *The Hatha Yoga Pradipika*. Woodstock, NY: YogaVidya. com, 2002.

Arora, Indu. *Yoga: Ancient Heritage, Tomorrow's Vision*. Minneapolis, MN: YogaSadhna, 2010.

Aurobindo, Sri. *Letters on Yoga*. Pondicherry: Sri Aurobindo Ashram, 2002.

Balkaran, Raj. *The Stories Behind the Poses: The Secret Power of Yoga*. London: New Harbinger Publications, 2019.

Ballard, Jacoby. *A Queer Dharma: Yoga and Meditations for Liberation*. Berkeley, CA: North Atlantic Books, 2021.

Barkataki, Susanna. *Embrace Yoga's Roots: Courageous Ways to Deepen Your Yoga Practice*. Orlando, FL: Ignite Yoga and Wellness Institute, 2020.

Bhikkhu, Thanissaro. "Upeksha." *Tricycle: The Buddhist Review*, December 2020.

———. "The Brahma Viharas—Head and Heart Together." *Tricycle: The Buddhist Review*, December 2009.

Bondy, Dianne. *Yoga for Everyone: 50 Poses for Every Type of Body*. Indianapolis: DK, 2019.

brown, adrienne maree. *Emergent Strategy: Shaping Change, Changing Worlds*. Chico, CA: AK Press, 2017.

Cheng-Tozun, Dorcas. *Social Justice for the Sensitive Soul: Engage, Serve, and Self-Care in a Changing World*. Minneapolis, MN: Broadleaf Books 2023.

Crenshaw, Kimberlé. *On Intersectionality: Essential Writings*. New York: New Press, 2017.

Cullors, Patrisse. "12 Steps to Changing Yourself and the World." In *An Abolitionist's Handbook: 12 Steps to Changing Yourself and the World* by Patrisse Cullors. New York: St. Martin's Press, 2022.

Curtice, Kaitlin, B. *Living Resistance: An Indigenous Vision for Seeking Wholeness Every Day*. Grand Rapids, MI: Brazos Press. 2023.

Davis, Angela Y. *Freedom Is a Constant Struggle: Ferguson, Palestine, and the Foundations of a Movement*. Chicago: Haymarket Books, 2016.

Deshpande, Sudhakar. *Yoga: Ancient Heritage, Tomorrow's Vision.* New Delhi: New Age Books, 1992.

Desikachar, T. K. V. *The Heart of Yoga: Developing a Personal Practice.* Rochester, VT: Inner Traditions, 1999.

Devi, Nischala Joy. *The Secret Power of Yoga: A Woman's Guide to the Heart and Spirit of the Yoga Sutras.* New York: Harmony Books. 2007.

Easwaran, Eknath, trans. *The Bhagavad Gita.* 2nd ed. Tomales, CA: Nilgiri Press, 2007.

———., trans. "Taittiriya Upanishad 2.2.2." In *The Upanishads,* 115–16. Tomales, CA: Nilgiri Press, 2007.

Emerson, David. *Trauma-Sensitive Yoga: A Practical Guide.* New York: W. W. Norton, 2015.

Feuerstein, Georg. *The Yoga Tradition: Its History, Literature, Philosophy, and Practice.* Prescott, AZ: Hohm Press, 2001.

"The Four Brahmaviharas?" *Lion's Roar,* November 19, 2019. www.lionsroar .com/buddhism/four-divine-abodes-brahmaviharas.

Gandhi, Mahatma. *Non-Violent Resistance (Satyagraha).* New York: Schocken Books, 1961.

Goenka, S. N. *The Discourse Summaries.* Onalaska, WI: Pariyatti Publishing, 2003.

Griffith, Ralph T. H., trans. *The Hymns of the Rigveda.* New Delhi: Motilal Banarsidass, 1992. First published in 1896.

Harris Parris, Anana Johari. *Self Care Matters: A Revolutionary's Approach,* Self Care Agency, 2016.

Heyman, Jivana. *Accessible Yoga: Poses and Practices for Every Body.* Boulder, CO: Shambhala Publications, 2019.

Imani, Blair. *Read This to Get Smarter: About Race, Class, Gender, Disability & More.* Berkeley, CA: Ten Speed Press, 2021.

Iyengar, B. K. S. *Light on Pranayama: The Yogic Art of Breathing.* New York: Crossroad, 1985.

———. *Light on Yoga: Yoga Dipika.* New York: Schocken Books, 1979.

———. *The Tree of Yoga.* Boston: Shambhala Publications, 1989.

———. *Light on Life:* New York. Rodale Books, 2005.

Johnson, Michelle Cassandra. *Finding Refuge: Heart Work for Healing Collective Grief.* Boulder, CO: Shambhala Publications, 2020.

Kauanui, J. Kēhaulani. "A Structure, Not an Event: Settler Colonialism and Enduring Indigeneity." *Lateral: Journal of the Cultural Studies Association* 5.1 (Spring 2016), https://csalateral.org/issue/5-1/forum-alt-humanities-settler-colonialism-enduring-indigeneity-kauanui/.

Khalsa, Sat Bir Singh, Lorenzo Cohen, Timothy McCall, and Shirley Telles, eds. *The Principles and Practice of Yoga in Health Care.* Pencaitland, Scotland: Handspring Publishing, 2016.

King, Martin Luther, Jr. "Letter from Birmingham Jail." Southern Christian Leadership Conference, 1963.

Kraftsow, Gary. *Yoga for Wellness: Healing with the Timeless Teachings of Viniyoga.* New York: Penguin Compass, 1999.

Krishnamacharya, T. *Yoga Makaranda: The Nectar of Yoga.* Chennai: Srisarada Publications, 2010.

Krishnamurti, Jiddu. *Freedom from the Known.* San Francisco: HarperSanFrancisco, 1969.

Kumar, Satish. *You Are, Therefore I Am: A Declaration of Dependence.* Totnes, Devon: Green Books, 2002.

Lorde, Audre. *A Burst of Light: Essays.* Ithaca, NY: Firebrand Books, 1988.

Mallinson, James, and Mark Singleton. *Roots of Yoga.* London: Penguin Classics, 2017.

Maté, Gabor. *When the Body Says No: The Cost of Hidden Stress.* Toronto: Vintage Canada, 2011.

Nhat Hanh, Thich. *The Heart of the Buddha's Teaching.* New York: Broadway Books, 1999.

Nikhilananda, Swami, trans. "*Kena Upanishad.*" New York: Ramakrishna-Vivekananda Center, 1949.

———., trans. "*Shvetashvatara Upanishad.*" In *The Upanishads: A New Translation.* Vol. 4. New York: Ramakrishna-Vivekananda Center, 1975.

Noble, Donna. *Teaching Body-Positive Yoga: A Guide for Teachers, Students, and Practitioners.* Berkeley, CA: North Atlantic Books, 2017.

Owens, Lama Rod. *Love and Rage: The Path of Liberation through Anger.* Berkeley, CA: North Atlantic Books, 2020.

Paramananda, Swami, trans. *Katha Upanishad.* Bangalore, India: Vedanta Press, Advaita Ashrama, 2012.

Parker, Gail. *Restorative Yoga for Ethnic and Race-Based Stress and Trauma.* London: Singing Dragon, 2020.

Patel, Tejal, and Jesal Parikh. *Yoga Is Dead.* Podcast. 2019.

Prabhavananda, Swami, and Frederick Manchester, trans. "*Mundaka Upanishad 2.2.3.*" In *The Upanishads: Breath of the Eternal.* New York: Signet Classics, 2002.

Raheem, Octavia. *Pause. Rest. Be.: Stillness Practices for Courage in Times of Change.* Boulder, CO: Shambhala Publications, 2021.

Ranganathan, Shyam. *The Yoga Sūtras of Patañjali: A New Edition, Translation, and Commentary.* New York: North Point Press, 2014.

Roy, Arundhati. *Field Notes on Democracy: Listening to Grasshoppers.* Chicago: Haymarket Books, 2009.

Saraswati, Swami Satyananda. *Prana and Pranayama.* Munger, Bihar, India: Yoga Publications Trust, 2009.

Sarvananda, Swami, trans. *Maitri Upanishad.* Varanasi, India: Sri Ramakrishna Math, 2007.

Shankaracharya, Adi. *Bhagavad Gita with Shankara Bhashya.* Translated by Swami Gambhirananda. Kolkata: Advaita Ashrama, 1997.

Sinh, Pancham, trans. *Hatha Yoga Pradipika.* New Delhi: Munshiram Mano-harlal, 2004.

Sood, Sheena. "Cultivating a Yogic Theology of Collective Healing: A Yogini's Journey Disrupting White Supremacy, Hindu Fundamentalism, and Casteism." *Yoga and Race Journal,* March 2017.

Soundararajan, Thenmozhi. *The Trauma of Caste: A Dalit Feminist Meditation on Survivorship, Healing, and Abolition.* Berkeley, CA: North Atlantic Books, 2022.

Sovik, Rolf. "Yoga and the Ego." *Yoga International.* Accessed December 2023, https://yogainternational.com/article/view/yoga-and-the-ego/.

Sparrowe, Linda. *Yoga At Home: Inspiration for Creating Your Own Home Practice.* New York: Rizzoli, 2015.

Stanley, Jessamyn. *Yoke: My Yoga of Self-Acceptance.* New York: Workman, 2021.

Thoreau, Henry David. *Walden.* Boston: Ticknor and Fields, 1854.

Tigunait, Pandit Rajmani. *Patanjali's Yoga Sutras.* Honesdale, PA: Himalayan Institute Press, 2014.

Tuck, Eve, and K. Wayne Yang. "Decolonization is Not a Metaphor." *Decolonization: Indigeneity, Education & Society* 1, no. 1 (2012): 1–40.

Vaid-Menon, Alok. *Beyond the Gender Binary.* New York: Penguin Workshop, 2020.

Valmiki. *Yoga Vashistha.* Translated by Swami Venkatesananda. Albany: State University of New York Press, 1984.

Venkatesananda, Swami, trans. *Vasistha's Yoga.* Albany: State University of New York Press, 1993.

Vivekananda, Swami. "Addresses at The Parliament of Religions." In *The Complete Works of Swami Vivekananda.* Vol. 1. Kolkata: Advaita Ashrama, 1989. Originally presented at the World's Parliament of Religions, Chicago, September 1893.

Whitwell, Mark. "The Five Crucial Principles That Have Been Left Out of Yoga Teacher Trainings." Medium, February 14, 2023. https://markwhitwell.medium.com/the-five-crucial-principles-that-have-been-left-out-of-yoga-teacher-trainings-mark-whitwell-3b8f8a6add6e.

Williams, Justice Roe, Roc Rochon, and Lawrence Koval, eds. *Deconstructing the Fitness-Industrial Complex: How to Resist, Disrupt, and Reclaim What It Means to Be Fit in American Culture.* Berkeley, CA: North Atlantic Books, 2023.

Yamasaki, Zabie. *Yoga for Sexual Trauma: A Healing Guide and Workbook.* Oakland, CA: New Harbinger Publications, 2019.

Yogananda, Paramhansa. *How to Love and Be Loved.* Nevada City, CA: Crystal Clarity Publishers, 2002.

About the Author

SUSANNA BARKATAKI has been called "a trailblazing yoga leader and visionary for our times." She is tech founder of Yoke Yoga, a free yoga app of micro practices for more peace in seconds, bringing yoga socially to all people to help solve everyday problems. She also founded Ignite Institute for Yogic Leadership and Social Change, where she runs award-winning 200- and 300-hour yoga teacher training programs to train students in using authentic spiritual tools to create positive social change

Learn more at SusannaBarkataki.com, and join her on social media @SusannaBarkataki. She has prepared a supportive resource of practices from within this book for you; visit IgniteYourYoga.com to get these free resources.